T0143651

BASIC HEALTH
PUBLICATIONS
USER'S GUIDE

TO
WEIGHT-LOSS
SUPPLEMENTS

*Learn How to Sort
Through All the Fads
and Supplements
and Successfully
Lose Weight.*

DALLAS CLOUATRE, PH.D.

JACK CHALLEM Series Editor

The information contained in this book is based upon the research and personal and professional experiences of the author. It is not intended as a substitute for consulting with your physician or other healthcare provider. Any attempt to diagnose and treat an illness should be done under the direction of a healthcare professional.

The publisher does not advocate the use of any partic ular healthcare protocol but believes the information in this book should be available to the public. The publisher and author are not responsible for any adverse effects or consequences resulting from the use of the suggestions, preparations, or procedures discussed in this book. Should the reader have any questions concerning the appropriateness of any procedures or prepa rations mentioned, the author and the publisher strongly suggest consulting a professional healthcare advisor.

Series Editor: Jack Challem
Editor: Carol Rosenberg
Typesetter: Gary A. Rosenberg
Series Cover Designer: Mike Stromberg

Basic Health Publications User's Guides are published by Basic Health Publications, Inc.

CONTENTS

INTRODUCTION

Want to add three, seven, or even more years to your life? Want to reduce your insurance and medical bills? Want to add more spring to your step—and maybe to a few other areas, as well? How about improving your chances at getting a new job or that promotion you've applied for? For six out of ten Americans, there is a simple answer. Just lose weight.

Unfortunately, actually getting rid of the excess pounds and keeping them off for most dieters isn't quite so simple. Not that there aren't lots of products out there that claim to be magic bullets. You see the ads everywhere. "Promotes Weight Loss." "Incredible Energy. Rapid Weight Loss." "Weight-Loss Breakthrough of the Decade!" "Fat-Blocker!" "Thermogenic Wonder!" There are so many competing approaches that no one other than an expert can pick his or her way through the chaos. What the average dieter needs is a guide to why body weight matters, what causes weight gain, and the options available for getting leaner *and* improving health.

The first reaction of some readers to dieting issues will be skepticism: "Is there even a need for diets and diet products? The answer is to eat less, right?" They would not be alone. Until about a decade ago, cutting food intake was considered to be the principal method for losing weight. At universities and nutritional research centers around the world, this view is changing. A recent study at the National Institutes of Health suggests that there is no evidence that caloric restriction is a good long-term strategy for weight loss. In fact, for some people, cutting back on calories will lead to health risks.

Certainly, those who significantly overeat can benefit from reducing their caloric intake. In general, however, calorie counting is not the solution to weight problems. Many reduced calorie diets are initially effective for achieving rapid weight loss, but the weight is quickly regained once the diet is over because the pounds lost consisted primarily of water and lean muscle tissue. The result of the typical diet is that the percentage of the body's tissues made up of fat usually is increased and the percentage made up of lean tissues—the tissues that burn calories—is decreased! The energy balances in the body are upset and future diets become more difficult because the body no longer responds. This is why the typical diet leads to the "yo-yo" pattern of weight loss/weight gain, with each cycle of weight gain more extreme than the previous one.

A weight-loss program should not just take off unwanted pounds. It should help you to feel good *and* look good. And the results should last! The goal is to make changes in body composition and metabolism that increase the body's ability to burn calories. Modifying the foods you eat and the supplements you take can make all the difference as to whether you achieve your weight-loss goals.

Guiding you toward the diets, habits, and supplements that are right for you as an individual is the purpose of this book. This *User's Guide to Weight-Loss Supplements* is designed to remove the confusion that so often arises from the babble of claims found in the marketplace. It will lead you step-by-step through the issues and the available solutions related to losing weight.

Chapters 1 through 5 tell you what the risks are

in gaining excess pounds, why it happens, and how you can determine the weight that is realistically achievable for you. Although you may find that you must swear off the "ten pounds in ten days" programs, you will be pleasantly surprised to learn that some plans really do work. Chapters 6 through 9 give enough basic information on the ways our bodies work to allow you to understand the choices you need to make to win the "battle of the bulge." Finally, Chapters 10 through 14 give the skinny on the supplements.

CHAPTER 1

THE RISKS OF EXCESS WEIGHT

According to a 2003 editorial in the *Journal of the American Medical Association,* obesity has become pandemic in the United States. Today, two in three adults are classified as being either overweight or obese compared with fewer than one in four adults in the early 1960s. An astounding 61 percent of adult Americans are estimated to be either overweight or obese. This means that well over 100 million people in this country have crossed the threshold of increased risks for various health conditions.

Carrying excess weight is considered to be the second leading cause of preventable death in the United States. It increases the risks for all of the following:

- hypertension

- dyslipidemia (elevated cholesterol and triglycerides)

- diabetes type 2

- coronary heart disease

- stroke

- gallbladder disease

- osteoarthritis

- sleep apnea and respiratory problems

- endometrial, breast, prostate, and colon cancers

Ideal Weight

The weight range, depending on height and frame size, at which basic health is best and the risks of disease and death are lowest.

Believe it or not, this list still leaves out many conditions for which excess weight increases the risks. Merely being overweight by age forty cuts three years off of one's life; being obese cuts between 5.8 and 7.1 years from life expectancy.

Defining Obesity

At one time, obesity was defined as being roughly twenty pounds over one's desirable weight. This older definition obviously does not take into account how tall one is, the heaviness of the bones, and so forth. Therefore, the medical world adopted another definition based on the body-mass index (BMI), which is a measure of your height/weight ratio. Using this definition, someone is overweight if he has a BMI of 25 to 29.9. He is obese if his BMI is more than 30. There is a special category for individuals who are morbidly obese (BMI of 40 or more), which is to say, individuals who generally are at least one hundred pounds over their ideal weights. Determining your own BMI is not difficult if you have a calculator or computer handy.

WEIGHT RISK LEVELS	
Low Risk (Normal Weight)	BMI = 20–24.9
Moderate Risk (Overweight)	BMI = 25–29.9
High Risk (Clinical Obesity)	BMI = 30–39.9
Highest Risk (Morbid Obesity)	BMI = over 40

Calculating Your BMI

The hardest part of determining your BMI if you are not used to the metric system is keeping straight the fact that the measurements are not in pounds and inches. One kilogram is equal to 2.2 pounds.

One meter is equal to 39.4 inches. One inch is equal to 0.0254 meters. A common weight is 70 kg, which is 70 times 2.2 = 154 pounds. If you weigh 154 pounds, then you would reverse the procedure and divide this by 2.2 to get 70 kg. Similarly, for height, if you are 5 foot 10 inches, convert this first to inches (70 inches) and then multiply by 0.0254 to get 1.8 meters.

Now you are ready to figure your BMI. The BMI is calculated by taking your weight in kilograms and dividing it by the square of your height in meters. Using the weight and height above, this means that a person weighing 154 pounds and standing 5 foot 10 inches tall would first convert to the metric measures of 70 kg and 1.8 meters. In this case, 70 divided by 3.24 (1.8 x 1.8) to give a BMI of 21.6. Someone 5 feet 4 inches tall and weighing 150 pounds has a BMI of 25.7.

Is Weight a Matter of Culture?

There is an old maxim, "you can never be too thin nor too rich." For the most part, it does seem to be true that those groups that are better off financially also tend to be less likely to carry excess pounds. The obverse of this is the fact that until recent decades, obesity tended to be thought of as a condition that afflicts primarily minorities. Of course, there have always been important exceptions. Among Mexican-Americans, for example, the rate of obesity in boys rises with family income. Similarly, in parts of the Midwest, laying out a good table—and enjoying it—remains the tradition.

A study performed at Northwestern University a few years back found that Caucasian women tended to become obsessed over their weight if their BMI had reached approximately 25, which is the starting point for being overweight. African-American women, in contrast, did not view weight as a problem until they approached a BMI of 30, the demarcation for obesity. Hispanic women tended to similarly discount weight until they approached a BMI of 30.

Weight still matters, regardless of cultural expectations. The rate of early death from cardiovascular disease is about four times as great in black women when compared with the rate in white women. Other causes of death, such as cancer, are likewise elevated along with weight.

It's Never Too Late

The benefits of weight loss remain even in those who have developed medical conditions. In a survey performed by researchers at the Pennington Biomedical Research Center, when patients with diabetes, elevated blood lipids, and/or hypertension lost from 6 to 10 percent of initial body weight, the costs for medication dropped to $61 from more than $122 per month. Needless to say, general health also improved.

For Successful Weight Loss, Look at the Reasons for Weight Gain

Weight-loss supplements, as is true of any other tools, are most successful when matched to specific needs. The next chapter goes into this a bit more, and the reader is urged to consider its points before jumping to the chapters that describe nutrients and supplements. To give but one indication of why this is important, consider that some people eat because they are nervous, whereas others eat because they are depressed, and yet a third group does not eat too much, but rather exercises too little. Finding yourself in this mix can go a long way to determining your level of success.

CHAPTER 2

WHY PEOPLE GAIN

Weight gain can be thought of as having three different aspects. The first is genetic. If most of the members of both sides of your family are heavy, then you might suspect that the propensity to be heavy is in your genes. This does not mean that you cannot do something about your weight, just that under certain conditions you can expect to need to be more careful in controlling your weight than many of your neighbors.

Genetic factors certainly are important in weight gain. However, no competent researcher will tell you that the genetic pool for Americans has changed the way that our rate of obesity has. Something other than genetics is at work, and it has had an impact across our society as a whole. So, our second factor is environmental. It includes changes in the food and changes in living habits that affect most of us. We can influence these factors as they affect our lives, but this takes a bit of knowledge and planning.

Third, there are those causes that are tied pretty much to what each of us does as an individual. Some of us exercise more than others, some eat less fast food, some are under less stress, and so forth. In other words, there are always factors at work that each of us individually can change that reflect how we personally shape our lives.

Factors That Affect Weight

• *Genetics*

• *Environment*

• *Personal Habits*

This chapter starts with an overview of why Americans are heavier today than they were forty years ago and then suggests specific supplements to match particular reasons for gaining weight.

Genetics

Genetic factors alone do little to explain why 25 percent of Americans were overweight in 1960 and more than 60 percent are overweight today. Nevertheless, your genes do determine your basic metabolic type. For instance, whether you will lose weight best on a very low-fat diet or a very low-carbohydrate diet depends to a certain extent on the body you inherited. Similarly, some people gain weight if they eat lots of dairy products due to their poor ability to digest lactose or problems in handling milk proteins. Tendencies toward blood sugar control problems, likewise, can run in families.

Geneticists tell us that diets suited to our overall genetic pool do have several things in common. Compared to the standard American diet, they usually have more protein, a very different mixture of fats than we eat, a lot more fiber, and very few simple sugars. The diets eaten by our healthy ancestors were richer in vitamins, minerals, and plant nutrients than is the modern fast-food diet.

Environment

We inherit our genes, yet we can still control our fates by compensating for weaknesses. Our environment is another factor that we "inherit," but we can compensate here, too, as long as we realize what the issues are.

Modern American Food

The food that you buy in the local store has changed quite a bit over the last forty years. Unfortunately, many of these changes are bad for maintaining proper weight.

- Fruits and vegetables today contain 10 to 50 percent less vitamins and minerals than in 1960. (Source: United States Department of Agriculture nutrient tables.)

- The ratio of omega-6 fatty acids (found in most vegetable oils) to omega-3 fatty acids (found in fish, flaxseed, and walnuts) is now between 10:1 and 20:1, but should be roughly 3:1.

- *Trans*-fatty acids, which are found in margarine and almost all processed vegetable oils, interfere with the body's ability to use fat for fuel.

- The modern American diet gets more than 25 percent of its calories from added sugars. The World Health Organization indicates that no more than 10 percent of calories should come from added sugars.

Antidotes to the Modern American Diet
- *Daily multivitamin and mineral formulas*
- *Omega-3 oils from fish and/or flaxseed*
- *Protein from whey or soy in place of sugary snacks*
- *Added fiber*

Sugar Sources
Beet sugar, cane sugar, corn syrup, dextrine, dextrose, dried fruit, fructose, glucose, grape sugar, high fructose corn syrup, honey, invert syrup, lactose, maltose, maple syrup, maltodextrine, molasses, saccharose, and sucrose

The Car

The Centers for Disease Control (CDC) has actually plotted excessive weight gain against the age of neighborhoods. What was shown is that the newer the neighborhood, the higher the rate of being overweight and obese. Modern neighborhoods are built to accommodate the car and may not even have sidewalks! As a result, exercise is no longer a part of our lives. Every individual needs to get at least the equivalent of thirty minutes of walking per day. Walk to the store for small items, for example, rather than drive.

Television

There is a direct correlation between the number of hours spent in front of the television and weight gain. Of course, many of us combine this favorite pastime with another—eating fast food. As one recent medical headline read, "picking up a burger and fries to eat while watching the big game or a favorite TV show may be a hazardous habit for many Americans."

Faster Food and Bigger Portions

Every survey agrees that portion sizes have grown steadily over the last forty years just as the number of meals Americans eat at fast-food restaurants has also gone up. The stomach takes a little time to signal the brain that it is full. However, fast food eaten on the run does not allow for this. Patrons at fast-food establishments can eat a full day's worth of calories in five to ten minutes and not even realize it. Eating in front of the TV also distracts from the "all full" signal. By the way, that extra large soft drink provides several hundred calories from pure sugar.

Fast food crowds out fruit and vegetables from the diet as well as whole grains and other sources of fiber. Only 20 percent of Americans eat the recommended five-a-day servings of fruit and vegetables. Here is the breakdown for changes in American eating habits (between 1977 and 1996) from a recent study:

- 93 more calories from salty snacks, such as potato chips, pretzels, and popcorn.

- 49 more calories from soft drinks.

- 97 more calories from hamburgers.

- 68 more calories from French fries.

- 133 more calories from Mexican food, such as burritos, tacos, and enchiladas.

Mealtimes

As life gets busier, schedules get out of whack, mealtimes included. After a long commute home, it may be difficult, for instance, to eat dinner at a reasonable hour. But eating late in the day sets a pattern for the body to store calories rather than burn them. Moreover, eating late in the day means for most of us that we do not want to eat breakfast. Of course, if we are running behind in the morning, that is yet another reason for skipping the first meal of the day.

Wrong eating habits have a domino effect. If breakfast is not eaten, the entire metabolism slows down. Far fewer calories are burned as the body conserves fuel. Even worse, some of those calories that are burned are pulled from your lean tissue. Plus, there is the compensation factor. Most people with weight control problems find that they are hungry at around 4 or 5 P.M., snack, then eat dinner, and yet—surprise!—are again hungry at bedtime. If you discover that you want a bowl of cereal before going to sleep, you need to eat more for breakfast and lunch.

Exercise

Whether for the environmental reasons mentioned already or for more personal ones, most Americans get less than thirty minutes of exercise per day. Seven out of ten American adults don't exercise regularly despite the proven health benefits. The trouble is, the body is made to be used. The adage, "use it or lose it," is absolutely true for most of us if we want to stay lean.

Stress

Stress can be a major factor in weight gain after middle age, especially "belly fat." There is actually

Hormone
A substance produced in one part of the body, such as the thyroid gland, that is carried in the bloodstream to other tissues, where it acts to modify structure and function.

a tie-in between stress and exercise, as well. Quite simply, exercise helps us handle the effects of stress. A primary result of chronic stress is an increase in the levels of the hormone cortisol, and it is this hormonal imbalance that leads to many of the other side effects of stress.

Work performed at the National Institutes of Health and elsewhere indicates the following:

- Greater than 40 percent of adults show adverse health effects from stress.

- Between 50 and 60 percent of lost work days may be due to stress-related issues.

- More than 75 percent of visits to primary care physicians are related to health conditions and complaints related to stress.

Stress-induced weight gain is not necessarily linked to overeating. Elevated cortisol cannibalizes lean body tissue, reduces blood glucose control, and causes weight to be deposited around the midsection. Individuals in whom stress is the chief cause of weight gain should strongly consider *avoiding* diet supplements that are stimulants. Instead, they might first try the alternative strategies given in Chapter 8.

Emotional Eating

"Emotional eating" refers to eating for reasons other than hunger. Mood issues are paramount. These include depression, boredom, loneliness, chronic anger, anxiety, tension, frustration, and so forth. Experts estimate that as much as 75 percent of overeating and binge eating has an emotional basis. Significantly, solace is not sought in protein foods, for which consumption remains largely steady under a variety of circumstances, but in fats, sweets, and other carbohydrates. In one poll done for the *Wall Street Journal,* ice cream and chocolate bars topped the list of mood-dependent food choices, followed in order by pizza, beer, soft drinks, hot soup, peanut butter, and hamburgers.

There are "triggers" usually associated with emotional eating. These can be social, emotional, situational, or even physiological. For instance, some individuals eat because they feel socially inadequate, but others eat to overcome headaches or pains. Whatever the trigger, keeping a diary of your eating habits can help to uncover it. Supplements for emotional eating primarily help to improve mood. A program is given in Chapter 8. Individuals taking any prescription drugs should always read the labels of supplements for possible interactions.

Seven Universal Strategies for Controlling Weight

Hunger is only one of the reasons that we eat. Often food is a way to relieve stress, a means to lift depression, or a diversion from troubles. Also, keep in mind that your body needs time to properly react to a meal. Mealtimes should be pleasant and relaxed, not hurried. To avoid eating more than you had intended—and more than your body needs—try the following strategies.

- Always eat breakfast and be certain to include high-quality protein in this meal.

- Eat more for lunch.

- Relax a bit an hour before the evening meal. Have an unsweetened cup of aromatic tea, such as chamomile or spearmint, and let yourself unwind.

- Have a bowl of broth or light vegetable soup before meals. Also, most people will find that their digestion improves if they eat a salad with the meal rather than before the meal.

- Whenever possible, fill up one half of your plate with lightly steamed vegetables, preferably green, and always eat the veggies! Do *not* count corn as a vegetable.

- Do not eat in front of the television set. This makes eating mechanical and tends to increase the number of calories consumed.

- Take a short walk a half hour after meals. As diabetics are taught, this little bit of exercise can help to even out the blood sugar response to meals.

CHAPTER 3

FINDING THE
WEIGHT THAT'S
RIGHT FOR YOU

Before beginning any program for personal transformation, it is a good idea to consider why this change is desirable and just what it is that you want to achieve. Losing weight is no exception to this rule. Good reasons include considerations such as health, beauty, and athletic performance. Bad reasons often mimic good reasons, but usu - ally bad reasons can be recognized as involving unrealistic expectations and other psychological reasons rather than health and a realistic view of physiology.

One of the most common unrealistic expecta- tions concerns appearance. TV and the press bom- bard us with images of "ideal" bodies, images of models and athletes, and so forth, but these are images that represent the natural body types of only a small percentage of the population—they are not most of us. Finding one's ideal weight means finding a healthful and sustainable weight that fits one's own metabolic individuality.

Physiologists sometimes divide all of us into three general body types, those of ectomorphs, mesomorphs, and endomorphs. These body types are inherited, although they can be influenced by diet and activities during the first two decades of life. Body types are rough guides to individual metabolic rates and to fat metabolism. It is not pos- sible for us to change our body types, and there- fore it is unrealistic to expect any program of diet or exercise to accomplish this feat. Dieters should discover what is realistic for their own body types and likewise discover the strengths that are the special virtues of each type. This is a much better approach than for all of us to attempt to be the same "ideal" person. The person who can win Olympic gold for distance events obviously is not the same person who can take away medals in either power lifting or Greco-Roman wrestling.

The following discussion complements the remarks in the previous chapter regarding why people gain weight. Just as not everyone gains weight for the same reasons, not everyone has the same natural constitution. Different body types are prone to weight gain for their own reasons. Eating too much sugar and *trans*-fatty acids will cause weight problems for almost anyone eventually. However, we also have our individual needs if we are to return to our proper weight.

Ectomorphs

Most people with weight issues idealize ecto- morphs. The ectomorphs are naturally slender indi- viduals who find it difficult to gain weight no matter how much they eat. Their metabo- lisms are fast burning and their abil- ity to convert food to fat is limited. Often they have great difficulty in putting on muscle tissue as well. Being an ectomorph may be great if you want to be a basketball star or a willowy fashion model, but it is not so good if you want to survive a winter in Siberia. Fortunately, most of us have central heating.

> **Ectomorph**
> *Body type that is relatively thin with long and slender neck and extremities.*

Can ectomorphs become obese? Yes, they certainly can. Typical ectomorphic cases of obesity may have been pencil thin in their early twenties or even later, but then they begin to gain weight rapidly. Ectomorphs are more prone than are other body types to psychological factors, such as nerv- ousness, worry, anxiety, and fear. To calm their nerves, they may overeat, and, especially, they may indulge in sugars and simple carbohydrates since these foods tend to encourage the production of the calming neurochemical serotonin in the brain. Also, feelings of security or stability may come with the added weight.

For these nervous types, calorie restriction is likely not the primary answer to weight problems. Rather, calming the excess nervousness, whatever its source, is the better solution. Whole grains and starchy vegetables can help calm the nerves without encouraging excess pounds, and various herbs and moderate exercise can be tried to reduce hyperactivity. This body type will also benefit from regular schedules for activities and meals.

Mesomorphs

Mesomorphs are your typical athletic types. They tend to be large-boned, more heavily muscled, and lean in their earlier years. Many of our champion bodybuilders are of this type, as, again, are many fashion models and actresses. Arnold Schwarzenegger and Jane Fonda come immediately to mind. Gifted with physical prowess in their early and middle years, mesomorphs are likely to begin to put on weight in later life as they slow down metabolically (we all do) and cease to be as active. Some of those most dissatisfied with their bodies after, say, age forty, are mesomorphs.

Mesomorph
Body type with sturdy, well-developed skeletal and muscular structures.

Weight gain in mesomorphs is most commonly the result of simple overconsumption. The appetite is good, so eating is satisfying in itself. The weight gained by mesomorphs often is much "firmer" than the weight gained by ectomorphs. Mesomorphs continue to have more muscle.

Mesomorphs often like the feeling of power and stimulation given to them by red meats and other concentrated proteins and also by spicy and fatty dishes. In the usual American cuisine, red meats contain lots of fat, as well as protein, and all these dishes are often combined with one or more relatively simple carbohydrate. Such combinations tend to have highly undesirable effects upon insulin production, and this leads to fat storage.

Mesomorphs tend to consume beer and other alcoholic beverages "to relax." Alcohol itself has many calories and it interferes with the metabolism of fat. Neither of these qualities is useful for someone who is overweight. If you are a mesomorph, take a hard look at how much alcohol you consume. It may account for 10 percent or more of your total calories each day!

As a rule, of our three body types, it is the mesomorphs who can most easily regain their proper proportions simply by reining in the consumption of excess calories if their weight gain has not gone on for too long and/or become too excessive. Unfortunately, true obesity, the gain of weight to something above 20 percent of one's ideal weight, tends to strongly derange the metabolism. Whether this is ascribed to the body's having established a new "set point" (either a brain- or a fat cell-mediated level of body weight) or to other mechanisms, once the derangement has taken place, it requires considerable effort to correct.

Endomorphs

Endomorphs are the third body type. These individuals put on weight easily and do not shed it readily. They likely have been what they consider "heavy" for most of their lives. If not too excessively self-conscious about their weight, these individuals tend to be somewhat more relaxed and calmer than the first two types. If their weight is brought into a balance appropriate for their body type, these individuals also tend to have considerable physical endurance and mental staying power.

Famous opera singers notoriously have en -

domorphic characteristics, but so did the great philosophers St. Thomas Aquinas and David Hume. Many professional football players display large degrees of endomorphy, but so does Marlon Brando. And what woman is not envious of the hair, eyes, and complexion of Elizabeth Taylor, who, again, has some strong endomorphic traits? Being an endomorph need not be a bad thing.

Endomorph
Body type that naturally has relatively large amounts of fatty tissue compared with bone and muscle tissues.

Endomorphic obesity often is related to a slow metabolism. This may be the result of inadequate thyroid production or of other hormonal conditions, it may be the result of the simple tendency toward inactivity, or it may be the consequence of the desire to have comfort, such as good food. The kidneys may be slow and there may be a tendency toward water retention for any number of reasons.

In any event, this body type does well by avoiding all simple carbohydrates and excess salt. Since there is already a tendency to store excess calories as fats, endomorphs do well to restrict all sources of concentrated calories. Bulky foods, such as raw and cooked vegetables, whole grains, and beans, are good choices, as are foods that increase thermogenesis. Aerobic exercise to speed up the metabolism is a great idea; excess sleep and naps probably should be avoided.

More especially, the amount of time spent in front of the television should be strictly controlled. TV watching has been shown to dramatically lower the metabolism for many individuals. The amount of time spent in front of the television is the second best predictor of obesity known!

The Weight That Is Right for You

These three body types respond differently to the same diets, and even at their ideal weights, they will never look the same. And why should they?

Most of us have bodies that are combinations of ectomorphy, mesomorphy, and endomorphy in varying degrees. Each of us can obtain her or his own ideal weight, but it must match the body each of us has.

Your ideal weight, as already has been indicated, depends upon a number of factors. However, the two most important of these are the size and density of your bones, and the ratio of lean tissue to fat stores. Weight charts have difficulty accurately placing individuals by bone weight, relying on visible features such as describing people as having small, medium, and large frames.

Likewise, the ratio of lean to fat tissues is best measured medically by the displacement of water in a test of underwater weighing to yield a result known as the body's specific gravity. Often the first stage of weight gain involves no gain of weight at all, but rather the loss of muscle tissue and its displacement by fat tissue. This shows up as a change in the specific gravity of the body. Only after the metabolism has begun to slow because of the loss of the energy-burning muscle does the individual begin to markedly put on weight and then find this weight difficult to remove. The moral is that scale weight taken by itself is less significant than is normally assumed.

Studies have shown that dieters are more successful by far in achieving a desirable weight and in maintaining that weight if they have an ideal weight clearly in mind. Therefore, readers might try this suggestion from *The Endocrine Control Diet:* One rule of thumb that has been used for determining ideal body weight for men is 106 pounds for the first 5 feet of height and 6 pounds for each inch after 5 feet, plus or minus 10 percent according to frame size. The rule for women is 100 pounds for the first five feet, and 5 pounds per inch thereafter, with the same adjustment for frame size.

Using this way of determining ideal weight, a

woman who is 5 feet 7 inches tall would weigh 100 pounds plus 7 x 5 = 35 pounds for a total of 135 pounds. Then factor in the 10 percent. A woman with a small frame could subtract as much as 13 pounds, whereas a woman with a large frame or any woman who is very athletic with heavy bones and considerable additional muscle might add as much as 13 pounds. So, the ideal range for a woman of this height can vary between 122 pounds and 148 pounds.

CHAPTER 4

ABOUT THOSE DIETS . . .

Most diets fail because they depend primarily upon reducing the number of calories consumed. Yet research proves that low-calorie diets are not the solution to lasting weight loss. Almost every dieter knows from experience that restricting calories very quickly reduces energy levels despite the initial weight loss common with low-calorie diets.

Did you know that on a daily diet of 1,000 calories, the metabolism begins to slow down within two or three days? Your resting metabolism—the amount of energy your body requires even when you are asleep—uses 75 percent of all the calories you burn in a given twenty-four hour period and is reduced between 10 and 20 percent on most low-calorie diets. Since your metabolism is designed to protect you against famine, your body will always defend itself against any large reduction in calories. Starvation diets fail to continue to produce rapid weight loss after two or three weeks as the body compensates. The dieter's dilemma is that with low-calorie diets you must cut calories to lose weight, yet cutting calories itself slows the calorie-burning process.

The weight lost on low-calorie diets consists almost entirely of water, and the rapid weight loss of the first few weeks stops as one hits a "plateau." But this is only the beginning of the dieter's problems. After a low-calorie diet, the body's base metabolism, again, the amount of energy produced at rest, will remain depressed for several months. Then comes the "yo-yo" or rebound effect as the pounds return—with a vengeance! Low-calorie diets promote fat storage, not fat burning. As for lean tissue, 30 percent or more of the weight lost on conventional diets is lean tissue.

Calories Sources

• *Protein: 4 calories per gram*
• *Carbohydrate: 4 calories per gram*
• *Fat: 9 calories per gram*
• *Alcohol: 7 calories per gram*

The Diet Wars

A variety of diets has been promoted as ways for dieters to escape the dieting dilemma. Some sort of diet needs to be adopted because we Americans tend to underestimate how many calories we eat by a whopping 25 percent! Nevertheless, most dieters are confused by so many diets making the same claims for what appear to be diametrically opposed eating plans.

On the one side, there are the extremely low-fat diets such as the one first popularized by Nathan Pritikin. The low-fat diets often get only 7 to 10 percent of their calories from fat, 10 percent from protein, and the other 80 percent from complex carbohydrates. Many dieters—by no means all—rapidly lose weight on such a diet. In reality, this eating plan turns out to be very low in calories as well as being low in fat. It certainly can be extremely hard to stick to for any period of time.

At the other extreme is the Atkins Diet. During the "induction" phase, carbohydrates may be limited to 20 grams per day, which is to say only 80 calories. Aside from this restriction, the dieter can eat as much protein and fat as desired. Critics point out that during the early stages of the diet, there is a great loss of water weight. During the later stages, all of that rich and enticing food turns out to not remain so enticing and the consumption of calories plummets.

Metabolism
The totality of biochemical processes of the body or the pathway and fate of a particular aspect of activity in the body, such as the metabolism of fats.

How can both of these diets work? Or can they? Two factors explain why both diets can succeed, albeit not always for the same people. These connected factors are insulin response and metabolism. Insulin is the hormone that your body uses to store blood sugar, to store fat, to convert carbohydrates to fat, and so on. Metabolism, in this case, refers to how your body burns fuel for energy.

Insulin response is very important because it helps to regulate the body's choice of fuels and how much fuel is burned for energy. This issue will be taken up more completely in Chapter 6, the chapter that deals with Syndrome X. The point to remember, however, is that fat metabolism uses different pathways than does carbohydrate metabolism, and the body cannot easily switch between the two. The higher the percentage of all calories that are derived from fat, the more difficult it is for the body to respond to calories derived from carbohydrates. If most of the carbohydrates in the diet are complex and slow to digest, then this does not pose a problem. However, the American diet consists of 25 percent added sugars; 40 percent or more of the diet is typically made up of simple rather than complex carbohydrates.

Insulin
The "storage" hormone produced in the pancreas: removes glucose from the blood, inhibits fat burning, promotes fat cell differentiation and fat storage, and moves amino acids into muscle tissue.

Under standard American conditions, the body responds poorly to insulin. Because of this, more and more insulin is released to control blood sugar levels. This surge of insulin reduces the body's ability to burn fat for fuel and encourages the storage of calories as fat.

A calorie is a unit of energy. In the body, calories yield energy during the oxidation of food, a process that at bottom consists of the chemical reaction of carbon and hydrogen with oxygen to yield water and carbon dioxide. This oxidation supplies energy for movement, for warmth, and to drive other chemical reactions. A pound of body fat is the rough equivalent

Oxidation

The process in which an electron, the unit of negative electrical charge, is lost from an atom. An example of oxidation is the rusting of iron.

of 3,500 stored calories. Supposedly, eating just 100 excess calories a day will cause weight gain of about a pound a month and simply reversing the process is said to take off the added pounds.

What actually happens is that the body is constantly changing not just how much food is eaten by regulating hunger, but also how much energy is generated. Insulin is one of the principal regulators of both hunger and energy. The other principal regulator is the efficiency of the fuel chosen.

Low Fat versus Low Carbs

The very low-fat diets, as long as they also are very low in sugars and other simple carbohydrates, work for two reasons. First, they are bulky and tend to be filling while still being low in calories. Second, they improve insulin response. Remember, the amount of fat in the diet helps to regulate how much in - sulin is required by the body to control blood sugar levels. Fewer calories with better insulin response equals an improved ability to burn stored fat.

This approach works with high-carbohydrate/ low-fat diets only as long as these remain low-calorie diets, as well. Carbohydrates necessarily require the body to constantly release insulin. Therefore, even the best low-fat diets can cause some individuals to gain weight and to have increased blood fats.

The very low-carbohydrate diets also influence

insulin—by not depending on it. All carbohydrates ultimately are converted to glucose, blood sugar. If enough protein is consumed, it similarly is converted in part to glucose, but most of us cannot or will not eat that much protein. Fat, however, cannot be converted to glucose. Therefore, on low-carbohydrate diets, insulin does not play a big role. Less insulin means less difficulty in burning stored fat. As can be seen, both the low-fat and the low-carbohydrate diets thus manipulate the same hormone, insulin.

Because low-carbohydrate diets often do not contain lots of bulk, they depend on a mechanism other than bulking to control hunger and increase weight loss. This mechanism involves what are known as "ketone bodies." Ketones are created in abundance when fat is burned without adequate amounts of carbohydrates. These are metabolites or breakdown products of the incomplete oxidation of fats. One effect of ketones is a reduction in appetite.

Ketone Bodies
Carbon-based compounds pro-duced when fats are incompletely oxidized. Ketones are eliminated via the lungs and the urine.

A second effect of ketones is metabolic. Ketones are fats that have been incompletely burned. They are eliminated via the urine and the lungs as waste products. In one sense, they are "wasted." Perhaps a quarter of the energy from the fats has not been released, but instead is being lost. One common analogy is green wood and a smoky fire. On a very low-carbohydrate diet, the body does not extract all 9 calories from each gram of fat, but rather throws away a big chunk. This is another reason that people lose weight on very low-carbohydrate diets.

Which diet is better for promoting weight and fat loss? In one study, dieters following 1,200-calorie low-carbohydrate diets (25 percent of calories) for three months lost more weight than did dieters eating 45 percent of their calories as carbohydrates (22.4 pounds versus 18.9 pounds). Fat loss was also greater on the low-carbohydrate diet (17.8 versus 15.6 pounds). Both diets kept protein at 0.65 grams per pound of body weight.

One "downside" of the low-carbohydrate diets is that most individuals who follow them fail to eat adequate amounts of plant-derived nutrients. Inasmuch as it is plant foods that primarily protect us against cancers and many other conditions, this can be a serious failing. Very low-carbohydrate diets, therefore, may not be good long-term choices.

Low-fat and low-carbohydrate diets both can work. A special difficulty arises when the dieter tries to leave one of these restrictive diets and reenter the world of normal food. Unless the dieter is very cautious, there will be a major rebound in weight gain. For this and other reasons, Gerald Reaven of Stanford University argues for a Mediterranean-style diet that derives 15 percent of its calories from protein, 40 percent from fats (mostly monounsaturated), and 45 percent from carbohydrates (mostly complex, little or no added sugar). Reaven may have a point. After all, he is the researcher who invented the category known as Syndrome X (see Chapter 6).

CHAPTER 5

WHAT TO EXPECT FROM DIET SUPPLEMENTS

Diet supplements are nutritional substances that manipulate digestion, absorption, and metabolism to reduce appetite and increase caloric expenditure. Some of these nutrients interfere with fat storage or increase the use of body fat as an energy source. Others, through a process called "partitioning," convince the body to use most of the calories consumed to feed lean tissues and for energy rather than to add to fat stores. The appropriate use of such nutritional substances has resulted in weight loss and in the increased ability to prevent new weight gain by thousands of individuals.

Certain nutrients are key factors in determining the body's tendency toward obesity or leanness. A truly effective weight control program must address the issue of fat metabolism at the biochemical level. It must take into consideration not just calories, but also the many factors that can impair fat metabolism. By choosing to include these nutrients in the diet, we can gain a measure of control over our metabolism and acquire some say in how much our body gains or loses fat.

Keep in mind the notion of metabolic individuality outlined previously. It is not just the food eaten, but the nature of the person eating the food that matters. Restricting calories may work wonders for the individual who gained weight solely because of a bout of inactivity and excess consumption, but whose metabolism has not been otherwise altered by the excess. This is the case with some—not all—women who gain weight during pregnancy and just need a little help afterward in losing it.

Yet for those genetically disposed toward weight gain, for those who have gained too much weight and kept it long enough to alter their body's regulatory mechanisms, and for those who for medical or other reasons have put on and kept on excess pounds, counting calories is usually a humiliating and futile exercise that does little or nothing to remove excess weight. Energy requirements can vary 100 percent among individuals of the same age, sex, and apparent body composition, and even those with the same relative amount of lean tissue can exhibit unexplained variations of 25 percent!

Moreover, the body is not passive in the face of a changing supply of calories. It constantly modifies its own energy expenditures in ways that make nonsense of simple calorie in/calorie out equations. How can it be the case that the woman not losing weight on 750 calories a day is not restricting her food intake sufficiently?

A few supplements are good for everyone. Most dieters will find that improving insulin response is necessary for losing weight—but not necessarily sufficient for guaranteeing weight loss. This is an important point that applies quite generally to supplements. *Do not expect the supplements to do all the work.* Supplements are aids that allow dieters to roll back the clock. Only appropriate changes in exercise and eating habits can insure victory and that the changes stick.

Many individuals will find that they lose inches before they lose pounds. This is because the program is designed to support the development of the lean tissue that promotes sustained weight loss. Muscle weighs more than fat. Therefore, don't be a scale watcher! Instead, notice how dress and belt sizes go down while energy levels go up.

Diet supplements also allow dieters to tailor programs to their own individuality. Metabolic stimulants, for instance, are not appropriate for everyone. Human beings vary greatly in how they respond to programs and products.

Whichever supplements are used and programs followed, allow enough time for the chosen regimen to work. Above all, do not look for the "quick fix." Programs that claim to help you lose five, ten, or more pounds per week are actually promoting the loss of water and lean tissue. "Water pills" and programs that promote extremely fast weight loss never keep the weight off and usually lead to weight rebound. A juice fast will cause anyone to lose weight in large amounts and quickly with the caveat that the weight will just as quickly return. On a good program, most individuals will start losing weight during the first week, but some will not see true weight loss for at least a month. Weight loss should average from one half to two pounds per week until you have lost up to 10 percent of your initial starting weight. Almost all individuals reach a weight-loss "plateau" after they have lost 8 to 10 percent of their initial starting weight. For sustainable weight loss, plan on following a program lasting several months to be certain that you have stabilized at your new, lower weight.

IMPORTANT

Before beginning any exercise or diet program, it is important to have a thorough medical examination. If you are under the care of a physician or are taking prescription drugs, consult your doctor before using weight-loss products. Do not use weight-loss products if you are pregnant or nursing, unless you are directed to do so by a healthcare professional. Children under the age of adolescence (roughly ages eleven to thirteen) should be encouraged to exercise rather than be given a weight-loss product unless there is a valid medical reason for intervention.

CHAPTER 6

CONQUERING SYNDROME X

Okay, we all know how much people dislike taking tests, but let's take a quick quiz that is relevant to anyone looking to lose weight.

What condition only recently recognized by the medical profession is described by all of the following statements?

a) afflicts almost one-third of Americans

b) is linked to obesity and weight gain

c) is associated with diabetes

d) is associated with high blood pressure

e) is a common factor in cardiovascular disease and stroke

f) is a primary cause of a lowered metabolism and fatigue

If you said Syndrome X, you go to the head of the class. The term "Syndrome X" is actually a description for insulin resistance and all the potential pathologies that can come with it (that is, obesity, reduced metabolism, cardiovascular disease, and so on). The term "Syndrome X" was dubbed as such in 1988 because insulin resistance is found

Atherosclerosis
Disease of the arteries in which plaques develop as oxidized fats penetrate the vessel walls and lead to progressive damage. When extensive, these plaques can narrow or even completely obstruct the arteries and cut off the flow of blood.

along with so many different medical conditions. In other parts of the world, other names are sometimes used. One such term is CHAOS, which is short for coronary heart disease, hypertension/ hyperlipidemia, adult onset diabetes, obesity, and stroke. Ouch! Another term for the same syndrome is insulin resistance metabolic syndrome (IRMS). The current medical favorite is "metabolic syndrome."

Insulin Out of Control

All over the world the scientific and medical community is starting to see that many seemingly unrelated diseases, in fact, are linked to a malfunction in insulin and/or blood sugar metabolism. Insulin resistance can underlie these various illnesses because the hormone insulin plays such an important and pivotal role in the body. Among the hundreds of different functions, the body uses the hormone insulin to control the amount of sugar found in the blood, to help pull amino acids into the cells, and to turn on protein synthesis in lean tissues. It directly regulates the storage of body fat.

When normal amounts of insulin do not bring down blood sugar after meals, the body secretes more and more insulin until serum glucose levels fall—usually too far—and the person heads for a big energy crash. We have all experienced the roller-coaster ride of too little blood sugar—the blood sugar "blues"—as low energy in mid-morning and/or mid-afternoon. Sudden urges to snack at around 4 P.M. and 9 P.M. also are typically tied to wild fluctuations in blood sugar levels.

Insulin resistance has several possible causes, in - cluding the overconsumption of simple and refined carbohydrates and/or a lack of adequate nutrients combined with possible genetic factors. Of course, the heavy overconsumption of processed simple carbohydrates coupled with inadequate nutrient intake is a mainstay of the American diet. Conversely, and not surprisingly, diets and nutrients that reduce the amount of insulin required by the body also reduce the tendency toward excessive weight gain.

An insulin metabolism that is out of control will make a person gain weight because insulin is the primary hormonal mediator of fat storage. Insulin resistance increases the number of calories stored as fat.

But wait, things are even worse than this suggests! It turns out that insulin plays a big role in whether we produce our own fat from carbohydrates. And if we are making fat, we are turning off our ability to burn fat because the body does not make new fat and burn already stored fat at the same time. As if this is not bad enough, the more excess weight as fat a person carries, the more fat that person is making from the calories he or she eats and the less fat that person is burning. Finally, a poor response to insulin causes the body to slow down and thus reduces the metabolic rate. In other words, you burn fewer calories even while you sleep.

Sugar Increases Fat Absorption, but Reduces Fat Oxidation

Bad food combinations can really hurt! Remember, we Americans already consume 25 percent of all of our calories as added sugars. Moreover, fast food typically combines sugars and fats. For instance, the supersized soft drink (16 teaspoons of sugar!) usually accompanies the burger and fries.

How bad can such combinations be? Taken in a milkshake, 30 grams of the common sugar fructose increased after-meal blood fat levels by 37 percent compared with control subjects. Sugars eaten with fats increase the absorption of those fats because all simple carbohydrates increase the levels of insulin, the storage hormone. At the same time, sugars eaten with fats radically reduce the amount of fat that is burned for fuel.

If the fat that you do not burn for energy is stored, then the combination of sugar with fat is obviously a bad one.

Avoiding Syndrome X

Although some individuals are genetically more prone to insulin resistance than others, fate is not written in our genes. A small number of steps can go a long way toward protecting against Syndrome X. Here are the starters:

- Eliminate sources of refined sugars, including hidden sources of fructose and milk sugar.

- Avoid overcooked and highly processed carbo-hydrates—processing causes starches to have significantly higher glycemic index values.

- Eat more lightly cooked green vegetables.

- Reduce sources of omega-6 fatty acids (for example, corn, safflower, and soybean oils) and increase sources of monounsaturated fatty acids (especially olive oil) and omega-3 fatty acids, such as flax and very high-purity fish oils. (See Chapter 7.)

- Examine protein sources to avoid pesticides and hormones.

- Stop smoking and avoid excessive alcohol. Red wine (no more than two glasses per day) and small amounts of dark beer are okay. Other forms of alcohol have no proven benefits.

- Get more exercise. Exercise, such as walking for fifteen to twenty minutes twice per day, improves the ability of lean tissue to accept blood sugar and tends to reduce triglycerides while increasing HDL, the "good" cholesterol.

- Take up activities that exercise the muscles of the upper body and torso. We lose lean tissue with age. Moderate weight training to increase muscle mass may be useful.

- Reduce weight. Fatty tissues increase insulin secretion.

Reducing surges of glucose into the bloodstream after meals is very important for preventing and reversing Syndrome X. Increasing your consumption of dietary soluble and semi-soluble fiber with meals can do a great deal in this regard. (See Chapter 13.) Not only fiber, but also other items that delay stomach emptying after meals may prove useful in reducing post-meal blood sugar surges. This effect is beneficial both for preventing the development of diabetes and for controlling the condition once it has appeared. Items known technically as oral trypsin/chymotrypsin inhibitors will delay the rate of gastric emptying and thus reduce glucose and insulin levels after meals. This has been demonstrated recently with an interesting extract from potatoes that can be purchased as a diet aid.

Reversing Syndrome X usually will only slowly improve weight control. However, not reversing Syndrome X will torpedo any diet program. Therefore, the choice is clear.

Supplements for Syndrome X

- Multivitamin and mineral formulation

- Vitamin C: 250–2,000 mg daily

- Natural vitamin E (d-*alpha* tocopherol, *gamma*-tocopherol and mixed tocopherols): 100–800 IU daily

- Trivalent chromium: 600 mcg daily

- Magnesium (preferably as aspartate or citrate): 400 mg daily

- Manganese: 10 mg daily

- Zinc (preferably as monomethionine): 15–30 mg daily

- Alpha-lipoic acid: 50–300 mg daily

- Silymarin (milk thistle extract): 50–200 mg daily

- Crepe myrtle extract (sold under the name Glu-cosol™): 48 mg daily

- Extracts from one or more of the following: *Gymnema sylvestre*, bitter melon (*Momordica charantia*), fenugreek seed, grape seed and bilberry

CHAPTER 7

SOMETIMES EATING FAT MAKES YOU LEAN

With the current constant push to reduce the intake of fats in the diet, it is easy to forget that certain fats are essential for health. The essential fatty acids (EFAs) must be supplied from the diet. Other fats, although not essential, are powerful health promoters. Both essential and non-essential fats—also called lipids—are required for the absorption of fat-soluble vitamins and related nutrients.

The two families of EFAs are the omega-6 family based upon linoleic acid (LA) and the omega-3 family based upon *alpha*-linolenic acid (LNA). The essential fats make up significant portions of the nerve tissue of the brain and elsewhere. They are building blocks for the body's production of hormones (including the sterol hormones such as testosterone and estrogen) and the production of hormonelike signaling compounds (such as prostaglandins). The immune system is regulated by essential fatty acids and compounds made from them.

Lipid
A term for fats and oils. Lipids are found in all cell membranes and are used for both energy and hormone production.

The Omega-6 Fatty Acids

Gamma-linolenic acid (GLA) is an omega-6 family fatty acid nutrient. Under ideal circumstances, it is made in the body from the conversion of linoleic acid. GLA serves as a pre-

Omega-6 Fatty Acids
• Linoleic acid (LA)
• Gamma-linolenic acid (GLA)

cursor to the family of hormonelike substances or "activated fatty acids" known as the prostaglandin (PG) series called PGE-1. This means the prostaglandin family "E" derived from GLA. The PGE-1 family is involved in anti-inflammatory, anti-spasm, anti-infection, and similar actions in the body, including reducing the "stickiness" of the blood. PGE-1, in other words, is a family of "good" compounds made from omega-6 fatty acids.

Prostaglandin
One of a group of hormonelike substances active in a wide variety of tissues.

Unfortunately, there is also a "bad" set of compounds that is made from omega-6 fatty acids, as well. The second family of prostaglandins (PGE-2) made from the omega-6 linoleic acid involves the production of arachidonic acid, a fatty acid already abundant in the American diet. The PGE-2 series activates aspects of the immune and other systems. In excess, it leads to inflammation, menstrual cramps, asthma, heart disease, and many other problems, including obesity. These are all possible results of the chronic activation of what is known as the *arachidonic acid cascade.* Among its other duties, the PGE-1 family serves to control or to turn off the PGE-2 family.

Most of us need a lot more of PGE-1 and a lot less of PGE-2. However, Syndrome X turns this equation on its head. High levels of insulin strongly increase the production of PGE-2. At the same time, the same factors that produce Syndrome X act against the production of PGE-1.

Many factors can prevent the conversion of linoleic acid to GLA and from there to PGE-1. These factors include deficiencies of the vitamins B_3, B_6, C and biotin, as well as inadequate intakes of the minerals magnesium and zinc. Too much alcohol, too much saturated fat, the consumption of hydrogenated (*trans*-fatty acids) and heat-damaged fats, and many other dietary factors are involved. Moreover, many people (especially those who tend to put on weight) have difficulty in transforming linoleic acid into GLA simply because they naturally produce relatively little of the enzyme needed for this transformation.

The Omega-3 Fatty Acids

The omega-3 fatty acid *alpha*-linolenic acid is found abundantly in flaxseed oil, whereas docoshexaenoic acid (DHA) and eicosapentaenoic acid (EPA) are found primarily in cold-water ocean fish, such as salmon and sardines. Although they are closely related fatty acids, EPA and DHA have somewhat different effects within the body. EPA acts mainly to suppress the arachidonic acid cascade and to increase the production of anti-inflammatory prostaglandins.

Omega-3 Fatty Acids

- Alpha-linolenic acid (LNA)
- Eicosapentaenoic acid (EPA)
- Docoshexaenoic acid (DHA)

DHA has a larger repertoire of uses in the body. For instance, it acts as a ready source of EPA because it can be reconverted to EPA when needed. However, DHA is far more than merely a potential source of EPA. DHA is critical for the proper functioning of the nervous system. It also has a stronger effect upon blood lipids levels. Although EPA can be converted to DHA, the rate of conversion may be inadequate to meet periods of chronic and/or elevated demand. Therefore, supplemental DHA, and not just LNA and/or EPA, may be of importance for maintaining normal health.

As is true of GLA, the transformation of these fatty acids from LNA to EPA to DHA and then to their active anti-inflammatory prostaglandins can be blocked by diets low in minerals and high in *trans*-fatty acids. Hence, although flaxseed oil as a supplier of LNA may be the least expensive source of omega-3 fatty acids, individuals who need therapeutic levels of supplementation should strongly consider using concentrated sources of EPA and DHA.

There is considerable agreement that for most of human history, and certainly before the advent of cereal grains, the ratio of omega-6 to omega-3 fatty acids in the diet was 3:1 or perhaps 2:1. In modern diets, the ratio is at least 10:1 and perhaps as high as 20:1. An excessive intake of LA, especially on refined carbohydrate-rich diets, promotes heart disease, inflammation, insulin resistance, and autoimmune disorders. Modern diets tend toward odd nutrient imbalances: They are high in *trans*-fatty acids and too high in LA, high in refined carbohydrates, rich in preformed arachidonic acid, but low in omega-3 fatty acids and in minerals. As a result, the pathways to the anti-inflammatory and also thyroid-supporting prostaglandins are either underfed or blocked.

How Essential Fatty Acids Can Help You Lose Fat

A study conducted in 1979 illustrates the effectiveness of GLA as a nutrient promoting weight loss. In this study, thirty-eight individuals took GLA in the form of evening primrose oil for eight weeks. Of the subjects who were more than 10 percent above their ideal weights, half lost an average of 9 pounds while taking four capsules per day. Only five individuals in the group showed no weight change, and the four subjects who took eight capsules per day averaged a weight loss of 23 pounds.

One explanation of the effectiveness of GLA is that it appears to increase the body's level of brown fat, a type of fatty tissue that actually burns fats for energy rather than storing fat. Brown fat (brown adipose tissue or BAT) is very important for thermogenesis. (See Chapter 12.)

GLA also appears to be important for preventing Syndrome X and diabetes. For instance, a low level of GLA available during development in the womb predisposes children to the development of insulin resistance. This bodes ill for children of the current generation of mothers and suggests that we will continue to see an increase in diabetes in the near future.

Omega-3 fatty acids appear to improve insulin sensitivity, to increase the oxidation of fats for fuel, to promote thermogenesis, and to help reduce fat storage. Over a period of several months, supplementation with omega-3 fatty acids may improve thyroid functions. EPA and DHA supplementation (4 grams/day) with active diabetics for six weeks has been shown to improve blood lipids, although there was no benefit to glucose control over this period of time. In general, omega-3 fatty acids raise HDL levels. Unlike GLA, omega-3 fatty acids cannot serve as a substrate for the synthesis of arachidonic acid, which is a positive point.

Conjugated Linoleic Acid (CLA)

Conjugated linoleic acid (CLA) is a fatty acid nutrient that occurs naturally in beef and in many dairy products. The reason that CLA can be found in meats and dairy products is that it is made from linoleic acid by the bacterium *Butyrivibrio fibrisolvens*, an organism found in the intestinal tracts of some animals, particularly ruminants, such as cows. Not all meats and oils are sources of CLA, however. Pork, chicken, fish, and vegetable oils, for instance, contain very little CLA.

CLA was discovered in the mid-1980s by researchers who found that a compound in beef exerted a cell-normalizing effect. Further investigations indicated that CLA is an immune system modulator—it alters some immune functions and how the body reacts to immune stimulation. Experimentally, CLA has been shown to protect animals to some extent against some of the adverse effects of being injected with toxins or certain types of vaccination. It has demonstrated anticancer benefits.

Currently, scientists believe that CLA alters the way that fats are broken down and stored in various membranes and tissues. The ratio of saturated fats to monounsaturated fats in tissues is altered in a favorable manner. The effect of this change in the several species of animals studied is a reduction in food consumption, a reduction in stored fat, a better ratio of high density lipoprotein cholesterol (HDL, the "good" cholesterol) to low density lipoprotein (LDL) and total cholesterol, and a reduction in atherosclerosis.

The results of recent clinical trials with CLA have been mixed with regard to weight loss and Syndrome X. Although supplementation yields health benefits through the promotion of greater leanness, lower body weight in diabetics, and even anti-inflammatory effects, at least in males already experiencing Syndrome X, results have been slightly increased insulin resistance. This suggests that CLA might best be utilized for its virtues (promoting leanness, anticancer, and so on) in conjunction with other supplements that directly address blood sugar regulation, such as chromium.

Supplementing Fats for Weight Loss

GLA appears to be more important for improving weight control than the omega-3 fatty acids. It is found in significant amounts in human mother's milk, in the seed oil of the evening primrose plant, borage oil, and black currant seed oil. Doses from 90 mg to more than 400 mg of GLA have proven effective. This is the amount of GLA found in two to eight 500-mg capsules of evening primrose seed oil. Some individuals may find that they receive benefits only at the higher dosage range. GLA is often more effective when taken in conjunction with vitamin B_6 and vitamin E. *Because in modern Western diets, omega-3 fatty acids are almost always underrepresented and GLA (an omega-6 fatty acid) will do nothing to correct this imbalance, dieters should supplement with 2–3 grams of high-potency/high-purity omega-3 fatty acids from fish oil each day (500–1,000 mg with each meal) and/or adding flaxseed oil (1–2 tablespoons) to the diet.* Ground or cracked flaxseed supplies lignans and other healthful ingredients, but should not be consumed in amounts greater than 4 tablespoons per day inasmuch as an excess will reduce thyroid hormone function.

GLA has been reported to give rise to occasional mild acne. In the experience of one clinical weight-loss physician, large doses given to improve weight loss also may lead to increased susceptibility to bruising in a small number of individuals. GLA and the omega-3 fatty acids are polyunsaturated fatty acids and therefore need protection against oxidation and free-radical damage. They should be taken together with natural vitamin E (200–800 IU), grape seed extract polyphenols (100–300 mg), and/or *alpha*-lipoic acid (50–300 mg) daily. Concurrent intake of omega-3 fatty acids plus broad-spectrum antioxidant and vitamin/mineral supplementation helps to prevent GLA from being transformed into arachidonic acid and the "bad" prostaglandins.

Individuals who are taking prescribed blood thinners should consult their doctors before adding these essential fatty acids to the diet in any quantity. As indicated above, both GLA and the omega-3 fatty acids act as natural blood thinners and anticoagulants. It is in part because of the imbalance in and lack of essential fatty acids in the American diet that blood-thinning medications are so commonly required.

- GLA: 90–500 mg daily in divided doses with meals

- EPA+DHA combination: 1,000–3,000 mg daily in divided doses with meals

- Flaxseed oil: 1–3 tablespoons daily

- CLA: 1,500–3,000 mg daily in divided doses with meals

CHAPTER 8

REDUCING STRESS
IN THE BATTLE
OF THE BULGE

Can stress cause weight gain? Well, in a 1986 Dutch study, men who experienced many life events in a short period of time—one definition of stress—gained weight. This study also showed the importance of identifying and treating the problem (stress) rather than the symptom (weight gain). In these men, the excessive weight had disappeared in almost all subgroups a year later. The exception was the subgroup that had tried to lose weight by dieting. The men who had dieted had gained yet more weight.

Stress is a common human experience. It is more than just being uptight or having a bad day. It is a physiological imbalance that results in biochemical damage at a cellular level. Stress occurs when the body is expending energy faster than it can be regenerated. The body's stress axis is a system for handling emergencies. Or, at least, it should be.

This, of course, is the root of the problem in modern life. The body's stress system was originally created to help us deal with life-threatening situations such as the threat of a saber tooth tiger, a forest fire, an earthquake, or an avalanche. This biological response was designed to be short-lived, a "fight-or-flight" response.

Because the stress response burns nutrients and reserves at a no-holds-barred pace, it was never designed for long-term implementation. Moreover, because it was developed to deal with physical threats, although it might be exhausting, the fight-

or-flight response was meant to release physical tension. But what happens when the threat is not physical and the response cannot lead to a physical release? What happens when we are faced not with a tiger, but with mortgage payments, birthdays, deadlines for book editors, crazy drivers, and the like? Our primitive response to stress has remained unchanged. Civilization has not.

Our individual capacities to adapt and deal with stress are different. Much stress is generated through an emotional response that is expressed– or, worse yet, repressed. Aggression, impatience, anger, anxiety, and fear are all emotions that kindle the body's stress response. Following a fast-food diet, drinking alcohol, smoking, taking drugs, and so on further contribute to our physiological and biochemical strain. Stress only truly becomes harmful when we can no longer control our responses to it. Not surprisingly, an unhealthy stress response is often tied to emotional triggers. Both can play large roles in weight gain.

Cortisol, the Enemy

Stress, a mental term, is mirrored in the body by the release of the hormone cortisol (one of the glucocorticoids). Traditional allopathic medicine has not paid much attention to cortisol's overall effects on the body because it is very difficult to measure accurately and the timing of release often is more important than the levels found in, say, the blood. Only quite recently has a popular market book appeared that has made the issue of stress its core analysis for why individuals gain weight in their middle years.

Glucocorticoids
One of the corticosteroid hormones produced primarily in the adrenal glands and involved in responses to stress, daily metabolic cycles, and numerous other functions.

Our ability to handle physical and mental stress declines as we age. In fact, much of what we think of as a decline in the ability to handle stress seems to be an aspect of aging itself. Glucocorticoid levels typically increase and/or become markedly dysregulated as humans age. They remain chronically elevated and/or dysregulated in comparison with the levels found in young adults. According to various studies, a significant increase of serum cortisol levels during evening and night is found in elderly subjects when compared to young control subjects. Similarly, the rhythm of cortisol release is significantly affected by age.

Impaired glucose uptake and utilization by the lean tissues—arguably the very core of insulin resistance—is one of the primary metabolic effects of cortisol. Therefore, it is not difficult to grasp the connection between elevated or dysregulated cortisol levels and Syndrome X. The result is what is sometimes called "central obesity" or the "apple-shape" in which most of the weight is carried around the midsection.

Elevated cortisol not only causes weight to be deposited around the midsection, but it also leads the body to cannibalize lean muscle tissue, the very tissue that burns the most calories. Moreover, although stress can induce hunger as an aftereffect, stress-induced weight gain is not necessarily linked to overeating. This means that the nearly 50 million Americans who suffer from stress-related weight gain will not necessarily benefit from diets based on restricting calories. It also means that individuals in whom stress is the chief cause of weight gain should strongly consider *avoiding* diet supplements that are stimulants.

As unwelcome as this news might be, any permanent solution to stress-related weight gain must include managing the stress. This means either avoiding the causes or finding ways of channeling the effects. Meditation, yoga, and increased physical activity are all ways of dealing more successfully with stress.

Emotional eating is often related to stress. Keep in mind that stress is a subjective response. What is stressful for one person may be exhilarating to another. Emotional responses are usually tied to an individual's past experiences, and this is one reason that "triggers" or activating situations are so important. As with stressful situations, these triggers need to be identified and either avoided or worked through.

Two items that are commonly found in the American diet can undermine one's outlook on life. These are caffeine and alcohol. An intake of roughly 700 mg or more caffeine per day (about five cups of coffee) is often associated with depression and mood swings. Caffeine causes short-term increases in blood sugar levels that can be followed by dramatic downward fluctuations. Consuming caffeine, in other words, is yet another path to the sugar "roller coaster" of energy ups and downs. Cutting out caffeine and refined sugars for as little as one week has been shown clinically to improve mood in many individuals complaining of depression. The consumption of alcohol before bedtime can have similarly distorting effects upon mood. This is because alcohol consumption interferes with the body's natural production of melatonin, and thereby disturbs the nature and restfulness of the night's sleep.

The following supplements may help. The first group is intended to be calming, while the second is designed more for elevating the mood.

Supplements to Reduce Stress Weight Gain

- Calcium and magnesium combination: 250–500 mg of each with dinner

- Inositol: 100–500 mg at bedtime

- Pantothenic acid: 200–2,000 mg daily

- Chrysin: 500–3,000 mg daily in divided doses with meals

- Kava kava: 60–75 mg kavalactones two or three times daily; avoid kava if you consume alcohol or take any prescription medicines

- Taurine: 500 mg twice daily between meals

- Theanine: 100–200 mg twice daily between meals

- Extracts of valerian root, hops, skullcap, passionflower, linden, and chamomile, singly or in combination (as directed)

- Chamomile tea

- Bupleurum and dragon bone formula, other Chinese herbal formulas

Supplements for Emotional Eating

- L-tyrosine and L-phenylalanine: 250–1,000 mg daily between meals early in the day

- 5-Hydroxytryptophan (5-HTP): 50–300 mg daily in divided doses between meals

- S-adenosyl-methionine (SAMe): 200–1,600 mg daily in divided doses between meals

- St. John's wort: 300–900 mg daily of a 0.3 percent hypericin extract in divided doses with meals

- Acetyl-L-carnitine: 500–2,000 mg daily between meals early in the day

- Vitamin B_6 (25–50 mg daily) may improve the effects

CHAPTER 9

GETTING RID
OF TOXINS

The presence of toxins in the body and the reduced ability of the body to remove toxins produce a number of fairly typical symptoms. Multiple allergies are one common symptom of a toxic load that is beyond the ability of the liver and other organs to clear or detoxify. Indeed, a large percentage of individuals who are overweight do not experience optimal liver function. This results from the fact that toxins and other sources of oxidative stress place an enormous burden upon many systems in the body.

Toxins can promote weight gain in a variety of ways. For instance, toxins can promote fatigue. Fatigue, of course, will tend to prevent individuals from getting the exercise necessary to maintain the proper metabolic rate. Fatigue prevents training the body to use fat as an energy source. However, there are other less direct ways in which toxins can lead to unwanted weight gain. In particular, toxins can cause a peculiar response by the immune system that can induce water retention and poor hunger control in certain individuals.

The Serotonin Connection

Some toxins come from the outside, such as pesticide residues. Others are produced in the body itself, for example, if the digestive system is not functioning properly. Whatever the source, one outcome can be hyperactivity on the part of the immune system.

Normally, the immune system protects us against outside invaders, such as bacteria and viruses. It also functions to rebuild the skin, remove worn out tissues, and many other things. Activation requires the presence of a "trigger" of some sort. However, the immune system is also partially set in motion by a feedback loop in which its own activities can serve as yet new triggers.

Bowel toxemia and other sources of toxicity thus can cause a continuous low-level immune response. This low-level immune response causes inflammation and excessive permeability, not just in the intestinal lining, but in many other tissues. The up-shot is swelling and the leakage of fluid into the tissues beyond what should normally be present. It is a source of water retention.

Immune responses, including from allergies, call upon the body's stores of the substance *serotonin*. Serotonin is a neurotransmitter that helps to regulate the appetite control center in the brain. Many diet drugs work by directly or indirectly manipulating serotonin levels in the hypothalamus. One consequence of a toxic buildup in the body and of excessive immune activity in response to toxemia is a reduction in the supply of serotonin available to the body to regulate food intake. Instead, serotonin is used to mediate the response to allergies.

Neurotransmitter *Chemical messenger released by the nerves to bridge the gap between nerve endings and to send signals in the brain and other tissues.*

In this schema, which is part of the "food-mood" connection that will be discussed in more detail in Chapter 10, serotonin is linked to food cravings, mood, and energy swings. The cycle goes something like this:

1. The afflicted person eats a food that triggers a low level immune response.

2. This immune response lowers blood levels of

serotonin (made from the amino acid trypto-phan), which is involved in inflammation and immune reactions.

3. A reduced level of tryptophan means less sero-tonin for the brain.

4. This leads to discomfort, mood swings, and hunger.

5. As a result, there are cravings for simple sugars and carbohydrates, in part because these cause the release of insulin, which increases tryptophan levels in the blood and serotonin in the brain.

6. There is now a temporary feeling of well-being.

7. Excess insulin results in a drop in blood sugar, which leads to hunger and low energy, plus the exhaustion of available precursors leads to a drop in brain serotonin levels, which leads to hunger and to a depressed or unpleasant mood.

8. The cycle repeats itself, now either to control blood sugar swings or in response to renewed consumption of a food trigger.

Detoxification

The body can be detoxified successfully through a combination of the right habits and the use of supplements. The following are accepted general guidelines suggested by several authorities:

- Drink 8–10 glasses of water per day.

- Eat a healthful diet with plenty of lightly cooked green vegetables (2 cups at lunch and at dinner).

- Consider an occasional modified fast of special foods to cleanse the system (consult a physician if you are pregnant or diabetic).

- Exercise for thirty minutes per day; this can be broken up into two fifteen minute walks.

- Use saunas or hot baths to eliminate toxins via the skin (consult a physician if you are pregnant or diabetic).

- Keep a food diary to identify offending foods.

- Get sufficient sleep at night and arrange for exposure to morning sunshine to reset your internal clock.

- Reduce consumption of coffee and caffeine in general, especially late in the day.

Supplements for Detoxification

- Multivitamin and mineral supplement

- Fiber: dosage depends on the type of fiber (see Chapter 13)

- Vitamin C: 250–2,000 mg daily

- Natural vitamin E (d-*alpha* tocopherol, *gamma*-tocopherol, and mixed tocopherols): 100–800 IU daily

- Magnesium (preferably as aspartate or citrate): 400 mg daily

- Manganese: 10 mg daily

- Zinc (preferably as monomethionine): 15–30 mg daily

- Alpha-lipoic acid: 50–300 mg daily

- S-adenosyl-methionine (SAMe): 200–1,600 mg daily in divided doses between meals

- Artichoke extract (15 percent chlorogenic acid, 5 percent cynarin): 500–2,500 mg daily with meals (do not use if gallbladder is obstructed)

- Silymarin (milk thistle extract): 50–200 mg daily

- Glycine: 1,500–3,000 mg daily between meals

- L-Glutamine: 500 mg daily between meals

- Probiotic organisms, such as *Lactobacillus aci-dophilus,* to improve intestinal health

- Charcoal: according to directions for no longer than one week at a time

CHAPTER 10

APPETITE CONTROL
101

The body is a mechanism that is constantly correcting its course to match the demands made upon it and the resources at its disposal. The regulation of the appetite is merely one part of the metabolic equation in which calories consumed must, over the long run, match calories expended.

Hunger Signals

All hunger signals can be divided between those that are generated in the brain and central nervous system and those which are generated outside of the brain and central nervous system. The central mechanisms are chiefly governed by the neurochemical messengers serotonin and dopamine. The peripheral mechanisms are chiefly governed by blood sugar levels and other signals of energy balance.

Central Nervous System (CNS)

Refers to the brain and the spinal cord. In hunger and satiety, a part of the CNS, the hypothalamus, is active as a central regulator.

This dichotomy means that hunger signals can be controlled by influencing brain neurotransmitters, by influencing the body's energy levels and energy sources, or a combination of the two. Ideally, both mechanisms work in tandem. Pharmaceutical appetite suppressants primarily manipulate brain chemistry. High protein/low-carbohydrate diets primarily manipulate (stabilize) blood sugar levels and, to a lesser extent, thyroid functions.

As already discussed, hunger sometimes is a bit more complicated than just needing to eat for energy. Judith Wurtman, a nutritional chemist at MIT, argues that carbohydrates tend to calm us and to provide energy while relieving depression. Reactions vary with individuals, but the calming response appears to be related to the ability of carbohydrates to increase the presence of the calming, mood-brightening neurotransmitter *serotonin* in the brain. The increase in blood sugar temporarily elevates mood in those with uneven blood sugar control. Serotonin also regulates the appetite for carbohydrates, hence the rash of diet pills that increase brain serotonin levels.

Adam Drewnowski of the University of Michigan suggests that the neurochemical link may be even stronger. Food cravings in some people may alter the level of *endorphins*, naturally occurring potent mood-altering brain chemicals that are similar to narcotics in their effects. Drewnowski's research indicates that many food cravings can be blocked by the drug naloxone, which in clinical settings sometimes is employed to ease opiate cravings.

In other words, hunger is not all that simple and once the body has become unbalanced, appetite control is not merely a matter of not eating. Most diets attempt to reduce only the consequences of excess hunger when this excess leads to weight gain. These diets do nothing to reduce hunger nor do they do anything to address its causes.

Satiety

Satisfying hunger and producing satiety, the feeling of having eaten sufficient food at a meal, are not quite the same thing. As is true of hunger, satiety is controlled partly in the brain through the satiety center and partly by mechanisms outside of the brain. Studies have shown that during meals, chronically overweight individuals take much longer to process satiety signals than do lean individuals.

The signal for having eaten enough does not get through to the brain as quickly or as strongly.

Signaling mechanisms outside the brain also may not function properly. For instance, during and after meals, carbohydrate calories that are not immediately used for energy are stored in your body in the liver and muscles in the form of a special starch called *glycogen*. As the storage capacity available for glycogen becomes filled, monitors in the liver send a satiety signal to your brain indicating that you are full. This is one of the ways that the appetite is reduced during the course of a meal. However, when we eat simple carbohydrates or if we develop blood sugar control problems or gain too many extra pounds, this control mechanism stops working as it should. Individuals who are overweight and obese produce only one-fifth to one-half of the glycogen produced by lean individuals. Therefore, the satiety signal that depends on glycogen is weak or absent.

Thus, satiety has a "central" component that acts mostly in the brain and a "peripheral" component that acts mostly outside of the brain.

Example of Increasing Satiety Via Neurotransmitters

Let's take one example to show what is involved in increasing satiety by influencing brain chemistry. We have met serotonin already. Serotonin, which is produced from the amino acid L-tryptophan, is the neurotransmitter most strongly linked to satiety regulation. The diet drugs fenfluramine and dexfenfluramine (now banned) specifically target serotonin release and reuptake. Several still-legal drugs do the same. Hence, a natural pre-

Peripheral Satiety Control
Refers to signals coming from the vagus nerve serving the liver and small intestines, pressure (fullness) in the stomach, energy signals, and other mechanisms acting primarily outside of the brain.

cursor to serotonin, such as 5-hydroxytryptophan (5-HTP), would appear to have potential to aid in weight loss.

Does it work? Absolutely, although the amount of 5-HTP necessary to influence weight loss via appetite suppression appears to be quite high. Several Italian clinical trials have shown that in dosages of 600–900 mg per day, 5-HTP over periods of five to six weeks without dieting can lead to weight loss averaging 3.1 pounds to 3.7 pounds. On diets restricted to 1,200 calories per day, dieters lost between 6.8 and 7.3 pounds in these studies. The control group taking only placebo lost 1.1 pounds during the six-week trial. Weight loss of one-half pound per week without dieting is not a bad record. However, at the 900 mg per day dosage level, 70 percent of the 5-HTP group reported nausea during the first six weeks of the trials. The nausea did not continue into the second six weeks. More recent trials with diabetic subjects also found benefit with 750 mg per day.

Individuals who would like to try 5-HTP for weight loss might want to combine it with L-tyrosine to prevent daytime sleepiness and to improve the production of the other appetite-controlling neurotransmitter, dopamine. Thirty to sixty minutes before meals three times per day, take:

- 5-HTP: 200 mg

- L-tyrosine: 250–500 mg

- Vitamin B_6: 20 mg

If there is any stomach upset, build up to the desired dosage over the course of one or two weeks. Reduce the tyrosine if this dosage leads to irritability or disturbs the sleep.

At intakes starting at about 200 mg 5-HTP per day, sensitive individuals may experience complaints such as sinus problems, stomach upset, headache, and so on—that is, symptoms of increased serotonin levels. Otherwise, the compound appears to be quite safe. Despite the apparent safety of 5-HTP, those using prescription drugs should be extremely cautious about adding this compound to the mix of items that they are ingesting. It is very likely that 5-HTP will potentiate in an unknown fashion and degree the effects of many prescription drugs that are prescribed to alter mood or help induce weight loss. Those taking tricyclic antidepressants, MAO inhibitors, lithium, fenfluramine, dexfenfluramine, Prozac, Zoloft, Paxil, or any similar drugs should combine these with 5-HTP only with the consent and supervision of their physician.

Example of Increasing Satiety without Brain Stimulation

A number of ways of influencing satiety do not involve messing with brain neurotransmitters. One of the most successful ways slows down meals so that the satiety signal has a chance to reach the brain and, at the same time, increases a sense of fullness in the stomach. The recently popularized "volumetric diet" promoted by Barbara Rolls of Penn State University is an example of a method for increasing satiety without directly influencing the brain. This diet advocates a bowl of light soup before meals and other methods for increasing meal volume rather than meal calories.

There are supplements that can produce similar effects. Fiber will be discussed in Chapter 13. However, not only fiber, but also other items that delay stomach emptying after meals may prove useful in reducing both post-meal blood sugar surges and appetite. Individuals who are faced with Syndrome X may find such supplements to be worthwhile because this effect is beneficial both for preventing the development of diabetes and for controlling diabetes once it has appeared. Items known as oral trypsin/chymotrypsin inhibitors will delay the rate of gastric emptying and thus can reduce glucose and insulin levels after meals. Meals also become more filling. This has been demonstrated recently with an interesting compound extracted from potatoes.

This inhibitor from potatoes when given to humans has been shown to elevate levels of a compound found in the small intestine called cholecystokinin (CCK). The inhibitor decreases food intake by 20 percent during an open-ended meal in normal weight subjects. CCK is a compound that is released in the small intestine and is involved in satiety. It can be given in purified form to reduce appetite, but the body rapidly develops a tolerance for externally supplied CCK. Fortunately, this does not appear to be the case with the potato-based inhibitor. Weight loss has been reported to take place at about a pound per week. Dieters should look for the wording "potato-derived protein inhibitor (PI2)" to determine if a product contains this active ingredient.

Other Supplements for Appetite Control

- Protein: 10–35 grams with little or no carbohydrate as a mid- or late afternoon snack

- L-glutamine: 1–4 grams between meals

- YGD herbal extract of yerbe maté (112 mg), guarana (59 mg), and damiana (36 mg) per capsule: 3 capsules taken thirty minutes prior to lunch and dinner

- Fiber (see Chapter 13)

- Trivalent chromium: 600 mcg in divided doses with meals

- L-tyrosine and L-phenylalanine: 250–1,000 mg daily between meals early in the day

- Vitamin B_6 (25–50 mg daily) may improve the effects

CHAPTER 11

BLOCKING FAT
AND CARB CALORIES

Commercial sugar substitutes that provide the sweet flavor without the calories have been around for a long time. More recent additions are the "starch blockers" that target the calories from everyday foods. Similar items are available for fats. New products have now appeared that work specifically to reduce the absorption of fat or to replace the fats usually found in foods. The best-known product of this type probably is a form of fiber called chitosan that directly binds fats before they can be absorbed. Of course, a natural way to reduce fat and sugar absorption by the body is to increase the consumption of fiber, especially from vegetables. This method is discussed in Chapter 13.

Fat Binders

Chitosan is an extract from the hard outer shells of shellfish. These shells are their exoskeletons. In Japan, this type of material was developed for use in water purification and other similar purification purposes, such as in the food industry. The principle is that there is a positive electrical charge on the chitosan that draws oppositely charged materials to it.

The same type of fiber was developed in Europe, and the principle of electrical charge was recognized as having a bearing on fat absorption. Fats and bile acids are negatively charged, and therefore are attracted to the chitosan and bound before they can enter the bloodstream. The makers of chitosan products claim that fats equal to seven to eight times the weight of the chitosan can be blocked in this fashion.

Chitosan binds liver bile acids, but it primarily binds dietary cholesterol and other fats. Chitosan thus is used to reduce the absorption of fat from the diet. In effect, it is intended to allow the dieter to follow a low-fat diet without actually cutting fat calories.

The results reported by the European supplier of chitosan were twice the weight loss found with the controls during the first two weeks and roughly another 5 pounds better weight loss over the next two weeks. Blood pressure lowering effects were also significant.

Chitosan may bind minerals found in the diet, as well as fats. Similarly, fat-soluble vitamins and other such nutrients are unlikely to be distinguished from cholesterol by chitosan, and therefore a deficiency in vitamins such as A and E and in nutrients such as beta-carotene might develop. Therefore, any dieter using chitosan-based products definitely should take a good multivitamin and mineral supplement daily at a meal other than when taking the chitosan.

Chitosan, to be effective, must be used in large amounts, which is to say, amounts similar to those that are effective with plant fiber sources. This is to say that although chitosan may have weight-loss benefits if ingested in adequate amounts, these benefits are not striking for what is, in effect, a fiber substitute.

Chitosan is taken at levels that vary to match the fat content of a meal. It is available in tablets and capsules. Directions will come with products, for example, one slice of pizza with 20 grams of fat might be balanced with 10 chitosan capsules. If in doubt, take more rather than less.

Starch Blocker

A product called Starch Blocker received a great

deal of attention a few years ago. Although the FDA ordered it to be removed from the marketplace, a new and more active form is now again being sold with somewhat more limited claims. It was determined that the activity of the original was not nearly as great as then believed. The new item, called Phase 2, appears to have solved the problems of the original. This starch blocker contains the protein *phaseolamine*, a compound that interferes with the digestion of starch. Phaseolamine is an extract of the white bean *Phaseolus vulgaris*.

The principle of the starch blocker is simple. All carbohydrates come in three forms. The non-digestible types are called fibers. Digestible carbohydrates are either complex—a category made up primarily of starches—or simple, which is to say, sugars. Most individuals now realize that the excessive consumption of sugars is bad for health; nevertheless, an elevated consumption of sugars is very hard to avoid in modern, processed diets.

Complex carbohydrates, including starches, are universally converted to glucose (sugar) before being absorbed. Starch is found primarily in grains (breads, pastas, cereals, rice) and also in potatoes, corn, and a number of other foods. Not only do these starches ultimately end up as glucose, in the highly refined forms we normally consume, they do so very quickly. In conjunction with the sugars already found in the modern diet, this presents a definite problem for carbohydrate metabolism.

Phaseolamine works by inhibiting the actions of *alpha*-amylase, an enzyme produced by the pancreas and released into the small intestine. When taken in sufficient amounts, phaseolamine can block the digestion of a significant quantity of ingested starch. Used appropriately, it can inhibit digestion and delay the absorption of several hundred calories derived

Enzyme
A protein molecule that increases the rate at which chemical reactions occur.

from starches. The benefit is not only a reduction in the calories absorbed, but also a reduction in the amount of sugar absorbed inasmuch as all starches are ultimately absorbed as glucose. Phaseolamine, therefore, is an aid to dieters and other individuals who desire to reduce their absorption of carbohydrates and to shift the diet's effective energy ratio away from carbohydrates and toward other energy sources, such as protein.

Relatively large doses may be required, as well, with phaseolamine if this item is to be used for maintaining what is effectively a low-carbohydrate diet even when carbohydrates are being ingested. One or two grams per meal of this active ingredient may be required, so the manufacturer's directions must be followed closely. Again, if in doubt, use more rather than less. Also, starch blocker blocks starch calories, that is, calories from complex carbohydrates. It does not block calories from simple sugars such as those that are added to soft drinks.

CHAPTER 12

ENHANCING THERMOGENESIS AND THE THYROID

Almost any individual who has undertaken serious dieting is acquainted with "thermogenic" products. Most such products are based upon the Chinese herb *Ma huang* as a source of ephedrine alkaloids or the use of synthetic ephedrine. However, there are other, safer ways of en - hancing thermogenesis.

How Thermogenic Compounds Help with Weight Loss

As discussed in Chapter 2, individuals prone to obesity often have lower basal metabolic rates (BMR) pound per pound than do lean individuals, and obesity itself promotes a lowering of the BMR. After eating, most people see a lasting rise in energy production amounting to 10 to 20 percent of their prior metabolic rate. For reasons not well understood, overweight women in particular do not experience this increase in heat production.

Thermogenesis

Thermogenesis is an increase in the body's production of heat energy triggered by nutritional and biochemical means, such as in response to meals.

Certain naturally occurring substances, such as ephedrine, speed up the resting metabolic rate, act as stimulants, and suppress the appetite. Caffeine and other members of the xanthine family have similar effects, and can be found in coffee, kola nut, guarana, tea, yerbe maté, and many other herb teas and foods. The seaweed known as blad-

Basal Metabolic Rate (BMR)

Also known as the resting metabolic rate, this refers to the amount of energy the body consumes at rest.

derwrack *(fucus)* activates the thyroid and has been used in Europe to treat obesity and hypothyroidism since the seventeenth century. Bladderwrack is less useful in the modern period now that table salt is routinely enriched with iodine.

Many of the substances listed in the section above on appetite suppressants also act to raise the metabolic rate. L-phenylalanine and L-tyrosine perform this function by serving as precursors to the neurotransmitters and metabolic stimulants epinephrine and norepinephrine (produced especially in the adrenal glands). High-protein diets, which supply these amino acids, will tend to speed up bodily processes in general. Since thyroid activators often produce results similar to adrenal stimulants, the thyroid is also important. It is of great importance (see Chapters 2 and 6) to prevent the suppression of the action of hormones that release fat so that it can be burned for energy.

The bulk of popular thermogenic products are based on ephedrine and caffeine combinations. This is because to get the most from ephedrine, caffeine or some other compound that performs a similar role, such as aspirin, must be added. The primary benefit of ephedrine-based combinations is a reduction in appetite. For most individuals, 75 to 80 percent of the impact of taking an ephedrine and caffeine product will come from appetite suppression. It requires high dosages of these products to cause a significant increase in the number of calories burned per day. These calories are used to produce excess heat, hence the adjective "thermogenic."

The downside, of course, is that ephedrine and caffeine make many people nervous, can increase insomnia, can elevate blood pressure, may not be safe for diabetics, and for some can be just plain dangerous.

Burning Calories without Ephedrine

Several approaches have been developed to try to keep the "burn" of thermogenic products while shedding the side effects. One successful approach uses an extract of green tea. As part of a weight-loss study, investigators measured the twenty-four-hour energy expenditure of ten healthy men receiving three doses per day of caffeine (50 mg), green

Catechin and Epicatechin

Examples of flavonoids, a class of active antioxidant compounds found in plants.

tea extract (containing 50 mg caffeine and 90 mg epigallocatechins), or a placebo. The authors of the study reported that treatment with the green tea extract was associated with a "significant increase" (greater than 4 percent) in daily energy expenditure. This means that merely taking the green tea extract caused the subjects to burn about seventy additional calories daily.

Direct stimulation from caffeine was not involved in this increase in energy use. The effect was not linked to the relatively small amounts of caffeine found in tea inasmuch as the subjects receiving amounts of caffeine similar to those found in the green tea displayed no change in daily energy output. Significantly, the men taking the green tea extract used more fat calories—approximately 10 percent more—than those taking the placebo. Green tea, of course, contains powerful antioxidants and is generally considered to be a healthful beverage.

Antioxidant

A substance that prevents or controls oxidation. An antioxidant more easily donates an electron (is more easily oxidized) than the elements of the body that it protects.

Another approach to increasing thermogenesis is to find a suitable substitute for ephedrine. Widely used at this point are extracts of the dried immature fruit of the bitter orange (*Citrus aurantium,* Chinese *Zhi shi*), including proprietary extracts that claim to include all five active compounds found in this fruit.

One study combined 975 mg *Citrus aurantium* extract with 528 mg of caffeine and 900 mg of St. John's wort for use with an 1,800 calorie per day diet. At the end of six weeks, the subjects taking the active ingredients had lost 1.5 percent of their starting body weight (about 3.1 pounds), a result that was statistically significant. These findings suggest that synephrine, together with the other compounds found in *Citrus aurantium*, may be somewhat useful in weight loss, but only if taken in combination with stronger items, such as caffeine. Other studies imply that thermogenic formulas based on bitter orange extracts give satisfactory results only if combined with moderate caloric restriction. Bitter orange extract may increase the thermogenic response to a meal by approximately 4 percent.

Not surprisingly, most individuals with weight problems have difficulty accessing stored fat for energy. L-carnitine is one compound that the body uses to ferry fat into the mitochondria to be burned for energy. Taken by itself, L-carnitine may not produce significant benefits in weight loss. However, recent research suggests that better results may be expected if some form of choline is ingested at the same time.

Finally, maintaining good health habits has been found to boost the number of calories burned each day. Taking a multivitamin supplement daily is associated with burning about 4 percent more calories every twenty-four hours.

Supplements to Increase Thermogenesis

- Multivitamin and mineral supplement

- L-carnitine combination: 1,000–3,000 mg of L-carnitine plus 1,000–1,500 mg of choline daily

- Green tea extract (standardized for 50 percent or more catechins): 300–400 mg daily supplying at least 90 mg epigallocatechins

- *Citrus aurantium* extract (6 percent synephrine): 325–975 mg daily in divided doses thirty minutes before meals

- YGD herbal extract of yerbe maté (112 mg), guarana (59 mg), and damiana (36 mg) per capsule: three capsules taken thirty minutes prior to lunch and dinner.

- L-tyrosine or L-phenylalanine: 250–1,000 mg daily between meals early in the day to increase the activity of any of the above supplements.

- Vitamin B_6 (25–50 mg daily) may improve the effects.

Increasing Thyroid Activity

One of the chief drawbacks of calorie-restricted diets is their tendency to lower the body's rate of energy production. In large part, this happens because the thyroid hormones are either released at a lessened rate or become less active.

An Indian herb may help. It turns out that this Ayurvedic herb, *Coleus forskohlii*, may increase lean tissue in the body by improving the release of fats from storage for energy and perhaps by improving the action of thyroid hormones. In a United States patent, a standardized 10 percent forskolin extract is described as increasing lean body mass.

Another special Indian compound known as guggul, standardized as guggulipid (25 mg guggulsterones per gram), has been shown to have a dramatic impact upon cholesterol and triglyceride levels, as well as being an aid to weight loss. When using Ayurvedic weight-loss formulas for a period of three months, non-dieting subjects lost approximately 12 pounds more than those taking a placebo. Trials using guggulipid alone without any other herbs indicated that as little as 200 mg taken three times per day before meals caused weight loss in overweight subjects. The effective dosage may vary if combined with other ingredients. These results were under non-American conditions. In the United States, guggul extracts appear to be more successful as components of more extensive formulas.

A good combination is guggul with various phosphate salts. The thyroid-activating and weight-loss stimulation of this combination is covered by a United States patent. The principal ingredients in this product are guggulsterone, phosphate salts, and the amino acid L-tyrosine (a building block for thyroid hormone and certain neurotransmitters). Phosphate supplementation has been proven in European trials to prevent the reduction in thyroid action and energy metabolism that usually is found with dieting. In a clinical trial, this patented product led to weight loss of just under 1 pound per week.

The mechanism by which the phosphate salts work has been explored. These appear to prevent the reduction in the conversion of thyroid hormones to their active form normally caused by very low-calorie diets. In one study, thirty overweight women participated in an eight-week slimming program consisting of a self-controlled low-energy diet supplemented with fiber and mineral tablets containing calcium, potassium, and sodium phosphates. Although there were no great differences in weight loss caused by these salts, during periods

Low Metabolic Rate
A risk factor for weight gain. A low ratio of fat to carbohydrate oxidation, regardless of the overall metabolic rate, is also a risk factor for weight gain.

of phosphate supplementation, the resting meta-bolic rate increased by approximately 12 percent in one group and 19 percent in a second group. No one holds that supplementation with phosphates alone induces much weight loss, yet it is significant to find that phosphates can prevent the thyroid downregulation typical of diets. Approximately 3 grams of mixed phosphate salts appears to be required for this effect.

Dieters, especially those who have been through the "diet wars" several times, should try improving thyroid functioning before opting for yet more stimulants. In addition to items such as guggul, keep in mind that the thyroid requires building blocks for its hormones. Increasing the amount of protein in the diet helps, especially the complete protein found in whey. Similarly, over a period of several months, the essential fatty acids discussed in Chapter 7 may help.

Supplements to Support the Thyroid

- Multivitamin and mineral supplement

- Mixed phosphate salts (sodium phosphate, potassium phosphate, and calcium phosphate): 3,000 mg daily, preferably in combination with other supplements

- Guggul: as Guggulipid, 200–500 mg two or three times per day before meals; a purified ex - tract supplying 25 mg of guggulsterones three times per day before meals

- *Coleus forskohlii* extract (10 percent forskolin): 250 mg twice per day thirty minutes before meals

- L-tyrosine or L-phenylalanine: 250–1,000 mg daily between meals early in the day to increase the activity of any of the above supplements

- Vitamin B_6 (25–50 mg daily) may improve the effects

Can Spicy Foods Boost Your Metabolism?

If you want to boost your metabolism, but would rather not take pills that may increase your blood pressure, there is a way. Adding a bit of spice to meals can accomplish more than just giving zest to bland foods. Spices can both increase total calories burned and help us to metabolize fat for energy.

Recent studies have shown that dietary red pepper, such as the fiery liquid that comes in little bottles, can significantly boost diet-induced thermogenesis and increase the oxidation of fat for energy. Similar effects can be achieved with a constituent found in mustard. The pungent principles in ginger also increase metabolism, but by different mechanisms. An added bonus is that all three of these spices improve digestion. A report in the press in 1999 described a study done at Oxford Polytechnic Institute in England in which dieters who added 1 teaspoon each of hot-pepper sauce and mustard to every meal raised their metabolic rate by as much as 25 percent.

Those who want to try the spice diet approach might take 1 teaspoon of red pepper hot sauce and 1 teaspoon of spicy prepared mustard during the middle of each meal. (Hot Chinese mustard is too strong for most people at this level of intake.) If the meal does not include ginger, follow the meal with a cup of ginger tea. However, do not eat this much spice late in the evening; raising your metabolism very late in the day will interfere with sleep. This approach is not recommended for those with ulcers and gastrointestinal tract irritation.

CAUTION

No strong stimulants should be used by those with specific health conditions, including (but not limited to) diabetes, epilepsy, heart disease, high blood pressure, kidney disease, liver disease, and neurologic disease. Women with fibrocystic breast disease should avoid caffeine and other xanthines inasmuch as these may aggravate this condition. Caution should be exercised in mixing sources of caffeine and ephedrine, or these two with L-phenylalanine, L-tyrosine, or yohimbe. Taken together in excess, these combinations can lead to nervousness, excitability, insomnia, and nausea. Moreover, long-term use of large amounts of adrenal stimulants may be undesirable. The potential for the development of psychological dependence and abuse of ephedrine products is very high. Individuals should carefully monitor how they interact with these and other strong stimulants.

CHAPTER 13

FIBER FITNESS

Fiber exists in soluble, semi-soluble, and insoluble forms. Insoluble fibers are those for which humans lack digestive enzymes, and therefore, do not break down significantly in our digestive tracts. Cellulose from grain bran, some parts of fruits and vegetables, and lignin from legumes are insoluble fibers. These fibers provide roughage to insure bowel movements.

Soluble fibers, which do break down under the action of our digestive enzymes, include pectins and gums (mucilages). About a third of the fiber in fruits, vegetables, and many legumes is soluble. Some grains, such as oats and barley, contain large amounts of soluble fibers. These are considered to be highly desirable fibers. Pectins have long been known to promote wound healing, to slow the absorption of glucose from the intestines into the bloodstream, to bind a number of toxic chemicals thus preventing their absorption, and to aid in the reduction of cholesterol levels through the binding of bile acids.

Hemicellulose has qualities of both insoluble and soluble fibers. Psyllium husks, the dried seed coat of the Indian native *Plantago ovata*, is perhaps the best of these. It acts as roughage and absorbs and removes toxins from the intestines. It also moistens and soothes irritated intestinal membranes.

Fiber Aids Weight Loss

It is now recognized that the addition of fiber to the

diet, especially soluble and semi-soluble fibers, offers many health benefits. Mixtures of sources of fibers of various types can be designed to work together synergistically to maximize their health-promoting properties. They act to regularize bowel functions, including the control of both diarrhea and constipation, to soothe irritated mucous membranes in the gastrointestinal tract, and to absorb various toxins and bacteria, which are then eliminated with the help of the bulking action of the fibers.

Emphasis upon the role of fiber in weight loss has once again become a topic of interest at the beginning of the twenty-first century because of the relative failure of reduced-fat diets to produce the hoped-for results. The bulk of the fiber itself gives a physical sensation of fullness that helps to control how much is eaten at a given meal. Whereas appetite is reduced directly by the bulk of the fiber, it is reduced indirectly through the delayed emptying of the stomach. Slowing the rate that the stomach empties gives the brain a better chance at receiving a satiety signal, as was discussed in Chapters 2 and 10.

Individuals suffering from Syndrome X benefit from the fact that the bulking action of soluble fibers significantly slows the release of carbohydrates into the blood from the intestines. This avoids, as well, both the energy lows and the surges in appetite that characterize the body's responses to excessive insulin release.

Just how important is dietary fiber in controlling weight? One study found that lean individuals eat about 50 percent more fiber than do those who are either moderately or severely obese. The amount of fiber in the diets of the three groups was estimated to be 18.8 grams versus 13.3 grams versus 13.7 grams, respectively. Other significant roles for fiber include the lowering of total cholesterol and the reduction of the incidence of colorectal cancer.

People who consume the most fiber have 47 percent less colorectal cancer and 66 percent less pancreatic cancer than those who eat the least fiber. Since colon cancer ranks just behind lung cancer as a cause of death, the protection afforded by fiber against this particular cancer is of considerable importance.

Fiber Sources

The preferred sources of fiber are the soluble and semi-soluble varieties. Pectin, guar gum, oat bran, barley, and psyllium seed husks are such sources. Some of the new fiber products made from citrus sources may also come under this heading of preferred fibers. Whole foods can supply significant amounts of fiber. Oats, barley, oat bran, and various legumes can be added to the diet on a regular basis to supply sufficient quantities of these fiber groups. However, if this is not possible, the more concentrated of these fibers are available in tablets, capsules, and powdered/granulated forms. Tablets/capsules or granules/powders can be taken an hour before meals. These dosages should always be taken with at least eight or more ounces of water or serious dehydration can result.

Two special fiber sources are often promoted for weight loss and blood sugar control. Fenugreek *(Trigonella foenum-gracum)* is a traditional plant that recently has become the focus of attention largely because of a fiber derived from the seeds. Although there are some benefits from unique saponins found in the seeds, the blood sugar regulating effect of fenugreek seeds in clinical studies is likely mostly due to the inhibitory effects on glucose absorption from the intestines. Results in diabetics have been promising.

Another item sometimes used is nopal cactus *(Opuntia streptacantha* Lemaire). The exact mechanism by which nopal decreases blood glucose is unknown, but it is a good source of fiber and

pectin. It is believed to act primarily by decreas-
ing glucose absorption in the gastrointestinal tract
when consumed in fairly significant quantities.

Supplemental Fiber

- Fenugreek seed fiber concentrate: 3–5 grams
  daily in food or water

- Nopal cactus concentrate: 500–1,000 mg taken
  with each meal

- Psyllium husks: 1–2 tablespoons once or twice
  daily in water

- Flax fiber: 1–2 tablespoons once or twice daily in
  water

- Modified citrus pectin: 1 tablespoonful once or
  twice daily in water

CAUTION

Fiber may bind nutrients and medications.
Therefore, supplemental fiber should be taken
at meals that do not include vitamin, mineral,
or other nutritional supplements. Alternatively,
the fiber should be consumed well before
meals. Plenty of water should always be taken
with dried fiber sources.

CHAPTER 14

EVALUATING CLAIMS AND PRODUCTS

Before we try to evaluate the claims made by various weight-loss products, we need to first get clearly in mind the major factors that determine weight. Weight management for those who are overweight usually requires three components: diet, exercise, and supplements. Of these, the normal diet is undoubtedly the most important. As we found in Chapter 2, the current epidemic of excessive weight gain, above all else, is the outcome of changes over the last forty or fifty years in the quantity, the quality, and the types of food eaten in this country.

At best, only 20 percent of Americans consume the "five a day" fruits and vegetables recommended by virtually all medical authorities as the minimum required for maintaining good health. This means that 80 percent of Americans consume too little vitamins, minerals, and fiber. Of course, 60 percent of us are already overweight and another 20 percent appear to be playing catch-up. Many experts conclude that correcting the diet and dietary habits, such as eating breakfast and not eating late in the day, accounts for two-thirds to three-quarters of success in taking off and keeping off excess weight.

As with an adequate diet, very few of us get regular exercise. Those who are charged with guessing about such things estimate that only 22 percent of Americans exercise regularly. This means that only one in five Americans gets the equivalent of thirty minutes of exercise per day. If diet accounts for, say, 60 to 70 percent of weight-loss success, then exercise may account for another 10 to 15 percent.

This means that supplements likely also account for 10 to 15 percent of long-term dieting success. Too often, we expect supplements to do all the work. This approach never succeeds over the long term. It does not work with prescription diet aids, its does not work with ephedrine and caffeine, and it does not work in the case of any other diet supplement.

Marketing machines, of course, always suggest otherwise. And it is certainly true that many individuals can lose ten pounds in ten days through a variety of means. Juice fasts, for instance, will cause almost anyone to lose massive amounts of water weight quickly—along with lean tissue, but not much fat. This lost weight, however, will not stay off. Moreover, each time such a diet is followed, the weight will come off more slowly and it will be replaced more quickly—and then some.

"Dieting may be the major cause of obesity."
—JEAN-PAUL DESLYPERE, PROFESSOR OF HUMAN NUTRITION, UNIVERSITY OF GHENT

How about those ads that show a bodybuilder who lost twenty pounds of fat in only fourteen days? Can this be real? In a word, "no." There is almost always a trick that is used to achieve such results. You take a person who is young, naturally very lean, and who works out regularly and place this individual in a situation in which he or she does not work out and massively overeats for four to six months. He puts on weight. At the end of this time, he goes back to his normal habits while he just happens to also use diet supplement X. Studies going back more than a century have routinely shown that individuals such as this, as soon as they stop the overeating and the enforced lack of activity, will see the weight melt away almost magically. Any product or even no product at all will work just about as well in these individuals.

The 60 percent of adult Americans who truly are overweight or obese cannot expect such results. In normal weight gain, each pound of fat equals about 3,500 calories. What does this indicate? It indicates that even if one could somehow target only fat loss—no water or lean tissue—losing a pound of fat is equivalent to losing the energy of not eating for about two days. In other words, losing even one-half pound of actual fat per week constitutes an achievement. Keeping it off for five years represents a marvelous success story.

Here comes the old adage: If it sounds too good to be true, it is. Sustainable weight loss— weight loss that stays lost—usually ranges from roughly one-half to one pound per week until a person has lost as much as 10 percent of his or her initial starting weight. Even the most powerful products employed without a reduced-calorie diet, when tested clinically by disinterested parties, usually produce an average loss of about five to six pounds in eight weeks.

When you evaluate a product and its claims, always ask the following:

- Are ingredients and amounts clearly indicated?

- Is the amount of each active ingredient the amount shown to be effective in clinical studies?

- Are there any clinical studies using the product?

- Does literature about the product address a "condition," such as belly fat, without ever addressing the issue of whether the product itself has been shown to be effective for weight loss?

- Are there warnings and cautions that apply to you?

- Are the claims for weight loss too good to be true?

INDIVIDUALIZING YOUR PROGRAM

More than forty years ago, Roger J. Williams, the discoverer of many vitamins, published a book entitled, *Biochemical Individuality.* Already in 1956, Williams was able to explain why:

- There is no such thing as the average person.

- Some of us can better detoxify chemicals and drugs.

- Some people are more prone to diabetes than others.

- Low-fat diets cause some individuals to gain weight.

- One person needs higher levels of nutrients than another to maintain health.

The intervening years have seen much of Williams's pioneering work confirmed. In dieting, as in other areas of health, each of us needs to select a program that matches our particular physiology, our habits, and our circumstances.

The first step is to return to Chapter 2. Look through this chapter to isolate those aspects of diet, exercise, and other habits that have led to your unwanted weight gain. For instance, if stress is a factor in your weight gain, then metabolic stimulants may be short-term fixes that, in the long run, make your weight problem worse. For answers to stress, consult Chapter 8. If wretched dietary habits are to blame—and you likely already know if this means you!—then Chapters 6, 7, and 9 may be of more help.

The second step is to decide on a realistic goal. Not the goal that is right for your neighbor, your daughter, or some fashion model, but the goal that is right for you with your body and your genes. Chapter 3 should help here.

The third step involves learning what you reasonably can expect from supplements (see Chapter 5) and whether you have one or more special conditions that need to be addressed. For example, conquering Syndrome X (see Chapter 6) will not in and of itself necessarily make you lean. Nevertheless, it is an absolutely essential requirement for getting lean and staying that way if you are insulin resistant.

Finally, do not be afraid to experiment. Give any set of supplements that you try a chance to deliver, which usually means a two- or three-month trial. Many of the supplements can be used together, but some are alternatives. Be clear as to which is the case. If after a good trial, a supplement does not work for you, try to find out why and, if necessary, use a different tact. It is, after all, your life.

SELECTED
REFERENCES

Anderson, RA, Cheng, N, Bryden, NA, et al. Elevated intakes of supplemental chromium improve glucose and insulin variables in individuals with type 2 diabetes. *Diabetes,* 1997 Nov;46(11):1786–91.

Andersen, T, Fogh, J. Weight loss and delayed gastric emptying following a South American herbal preparation in overweight patients. *Journal of Human Nutrition and Dietetics,* 2001 Jun;14(3):243–50.

Ayyad, C, Andersen, T. Long-term efficacy of dietary treatment of obesity: a systematic review of studies published between 1931 and 1999. *Obesity Review,* 2000 Oct;1(2): 113–9.

Bagchi, D. Beneficial roles of chromium, selenium, zinc and vanadium on Insulin Resistant Syndrome. *Journal of the American College of Nutrition,* 2001;20, 5:581, Abs. 79, 2001.

Barbagallo, M, Dominguez, LJ, Galioto, A, et al. Role of magnesium in insulin action, diabetes and cardiometabolic syndrome X. *Molecular Aspects of Medicine,* 2003 Feb 6;24(1–3):39–52.

Belury, MA, Mahon, A, Banni, S. The conjugated linoleic acid (CLA) isomer, t10c12-CLA, is inversely associated with changes in body weight and serum leptin in subjects with type 2 diabetes mellitus. *Journal of Nutrition,* 2003 Jan; 133(1):257S–260S.

Eaton, SB, Eaton, SB 3rd. Paleolithic vs. modern diets—selected pathophysiological implications. *European Journal of Nutrition,* 2000 Apr;39(2):67–70.

Grundy, SM, Abate, N, Chandalia, M. Diet composition and the metabolic syndrome: what is the optimal fat intake? *American Journal of Medicine*, 2002 Dec 30;113 Suppl 9B:25S–29S.

Harris, MI, Flegal, KM, Cowie, CC, et al. Prevalence of diabetes, impaired fasting glucose, and impaired glucose tolerance in U.S. adults: the Third National Health and Nutrition Examination Survey, 1988–94. *Diabetes Care*, 1998; 21: 518–524.

Hongu, N, Sachan, DS. Carnitine and choline supplementation with exercise alter carnitine profiles, biochemical markers of fat metabolism and serum leptin concentration in healthy women. *Journal of Nutrition*, 2003 Jan;133(1):84–9.

Howard, BV, Rodriguez, BL, Bennett, PH, et al. Prevention Conference VI: Diabetes and Cardiovascular disease: Writing Group I: Epidemiology. *Circulation*, 2002 May 7;105(18): e132–7.

Khamaisi, M, Potashnik, R, Tirosh, A, et al. Lipoic acid reduces glycemia and increases muscle GLUT4 content in streptozotocin-diabetic rats. *Metabolism*, 1997 Jul;46(7): 763–8.

Looker, HC, Knowler, WC, Hanson, RL. Changes in BMI and weight before and after the development of type 2 diabetes. *Diabetes Care*, 2001 Nov;24(11): 1917–22.

Madar, Z, Stark AH. New legume sources as therapeutic agents. *British Journal of Nutrition*, 2002 Dec;88 Suppl 3:S287–92.

Mokdad, AH, Ford, ES, Bowman, BA, et al. Prevalence of obesity, diabetes, and obesity-related health risk factors, 2001. *Journal of the American Medical Association*, 2003 Jan 1;289(1):76–9.

Preuss, HG, Jarrell, ST, Scheckenbach, R, et al. Comparative effects of chromium, vanadium and gymnema sylvestre on sugar-induced blood pressure elevations in SHR. *Journal of the American College of Nutrition,* 1998 Apr;17(2):116–23.

Riserus, U, Arner, P, Brismar, K, et al. Treatment with dietary trans10cis12 conjugated linoleic acid causes isomer-specific insulin resistance in obese men with the metabolic syndrome. *Diabetes Care,* 2002 Sep; 25(9):1516–21.

Rump, P, Popp-Snijders, C, Heine, RJ, et al. Components of the insulin resistance syndrome in seven-year-old children: relations with birth weight and the polyunsaturated fatty acid content of umbilical cord plasma phospholipids. *Diabetologia,* 2002 Mar;45(3): 349–55.

Schwartz, JG, Guan, D, Green, GM, et al. Treatment with an oral proteinase inhibitor slows gastric emptying and acutely reduces glucose and insulin levels after a liquid meal in type II diabetic patients. *Diabetes Care,* 1994 Apr;17(4):255–62.

Spreadburr, D, Shao, A, Essmann, MK, et al. A proteinase inhibitor extract from potatoes reduces postprandial blood glucose in human subjects. *Journal of the American Nutraceutical Association,* 2003;6,1: 29–38.

Woodman, RJ, Mori, TA, Burke, V, et al. Effects of purified eicosapentaenoic and docosahexaenoic acids on glycemic control, blood pressure, and serum lipids in type 2 diabetic patients with treated hypertension. *Journal of the American College of Nutrition,* 2002 Nov;76(5):1007–15.

OTHER BOOKS
AND RESOURCES

Bennett, P, Barrie, S, Faye, S. *7-Day Detox Miracle*. Rocklin, CA: Prima Health, 1999.

Challem, J, Berkson, B, Smith MD. *Syndrome X*. New York, NY: John Wiley & Sons, 2000.

Gittleman, AL. *The Fat Flush Plan*. New York, NY: McGraw-Hill, 2002.

Rolls, B and Barnett, RA. *Volumetrics*. New York, NY: HarperCollins, 2000.

Werbach, Melvyn R and Moss, Jeffrey. *Textbook of Nutritional Medicine*. Tarzana, CA: Third Line Press, 1999.

Werbach, Melvyn R and Murray, Michael T. *Botanical Influences on Illness*. Tarzana, CA: Third Line Press, 1994.

Willett, WC, Giovannucci, EL, Callahan, M. *Eat, Drink and Be Healthy*. New York, NY: Simon & Schuster Source, 2001.

GreatLife Magazine
Consumer magazine with articles on vitamins, minerals, herbs, and foods.
Available for free at many health and natural food stores.

Let's Live Magazine
Consumer magazine with emphasis on the health benefits of vitamins, minerals, and herbs.

Customer service:
1-800-676-4333

P.O. Box 74908
Los Angeles, CA 90004

Subscriptions: 12 issues per year, $19.95 in the U.S.;
$31.95 outside the U.S.

Physical Magazine
Magazine oriented to body builders and other serious athletes.

Customer service:
1-800-676-4333
P.O. Box 74908
Los Angeles, CA 90004

Subscriptions: 12 issues per year, $19.95 in the U.S.;
$31.95 outside the U.S.

The Nutrition Reporter™ newsletter
Monthly newsletter that summarizes recent medical research on vitamins, minerals, and herbs.

Customer service:
P.O. Box 30246
Tucson, AZ 85751-0246
e-mail: jack@thenutritionreporter.com
www.nutritionreporter.com

Subscriptions: $26 per year (12 issues) in the U.S.; $32
U.S. or $48 CNC for Canada; $38 for other countries

INDEX

9 781681 628844